The Science of Well-Being: Integration into Clinical Child Psychiatry

Editors

DAVID C. RETTEW
MATTHEW G. BIEL
JEFF Q. BOSTIC

CHILD AND ADOLESCENT PSYCHIATRIC CLINICS OF NORTH AMERICA

www.childpsych.theclinics.com

Consulting Editor
TODD E. PETERS

April 2019 • Volume 28 • Number 2

ELSEVIER

1600 John F. Kennedy Boulevard • Suite 1800 • Philadelphia, Pennsylvania, 19103-2899

http://www.theclinics.com

CHILD AND ADOLESCENT PSYCHIATRIC CLINICS OF NORTH AMERICA Volume 28, Number 2
April 2019 ISSN 1056-4993, ISBN-13: 978-0-323-67789-9

Editor: Lauren Boyle
Developmental Editor: Kristen Helm

Child and Adolescent Psychiatric Clinics of North America (ISSN 1056-4993) is published quarterly by Elsevier Inc., 360 Park Avenue South, New York, NY 10010-1710. Months of issue are January, April, July, and October. Business and Editorial Offices: 1600 John F. Kennedy Boulevard, Suite 1800, Philadelphia, PA 19103-2899. Periodicals postage paid at New York, NY and additional mailing offices. Subscription prices are $335.00 per year (US individuals), $627.00 per year (US institutions), $100.00 per year (US students), $388.00 per year (Canadian individuals), $762.00 per year (Canadian institutions), $200.00 per year (Canadian students), $446.00 per year (international individuals), $762.00 per year (international institutions), and $200.00 per year (international students). International air speed delivery is included in all *Clinics* subscription prices. All prices are subject to change without notice. **POSTMASTER:** Send address changes to *Child and Adolescent Psychiatric Clinics of North America*, Elsevier Health Sciences Division, Subscription Customer Service, 3251 Riverport Lane, Maryland Heights, MO 63043. **Customer Service: 1-800-654-2452 (U.S. and Canada); 314-447-8871 (outside U.S. and Canada). Fax: 314-447-8029. E-mail:** JournalsCustomer Service-usa@elsevier.com **(for print support) or** journalsonlinesupport-usa@elsevier.com **(for online support).**

Reprints. For copies of 100 or more of articles in this publication, please contact the Commercial Reprints Department, Elsevier Inc., 360 Park Avenue South, New York, New York 10010-1710 Tel.: 212-633-3874; Fax: 212-633-3820, E-mail: reprints@elsevier.com.

Child and Adolescent Psychiatric Clinics of North America is covered in *MEDLINE/PubMed (Index Medicus), ISI, SSCI, Research Alert, Social Search, Current Contents,* and *EMBASE/Excerpta Medica.*

Contributors

CONSULTING EDITOR

TODD E. PETERS, MD, FAPA
Medical Director, Child and Adolescent Services, Chief Medical Information Officer (CMIO), Sheppard Pratt Health System, Sheppard Pratt Physicians PA Clinical Operations Liaison, Baltimore, Maryland

EDITORS

DAVID C. RETTEW, MD
Associate Professor of Psychiatry and Pediatrics, University of Vermont Larner College of Medicine, Burlington, Vermont; Medical Director, Child, Adolescent, and Family Unit, Vermont Department of Mental Health, Waterbury, Vermont; Director, Pediatric Psychiatry Clinic, University of Vermont Medical Center, Burlington, Vermont

MATTHEW G. BIEL, MD, MSc
Division Chief, Child and Adolescent Psychiatry, MedStar Georgetown University Hospital, Associate Professor, Departments of Psychiatry and Pediatrics, Medstar Georgetown University Hospital, Georgetown University Medical Center, Washington, DC

JEFF Q. BOSTIC, MD, EdD
Professor of Psychiatry, Department of Psychiatry, Division of Child and Adolescent Psychiatry, MedStar Georgetown University Hospital, Washington, DC

AUTHORS

ZOE ADAMS, BS
Division of Child Psychiatry, Department Psychiatry, Vermont Center for Children, Youth, and Families, University of Vermont, Burlington, Vermont

EMILY ARON, MD
Assistant Professor, Department of Psychiatry, Medstar Georgetown University Hospital, Georgetown University Medical Center, Washington, DC

YANG BAI, PhD
Department of Rehabilitation and Movement Science, University of Vermont, Burlington, Vermont

EUGENE V. BERESIN, MD
Professor of Psychiatry, Massachusetts General Hospital, Harvard University, Boston, Massachusetts

MATTHEW G. BIEL, MD, MSc
Division Chief, Child and Adolescent Psychiatry, MedStar Georgetown University Hospital, Associate Professor, Departments of Psychiatry and Pediatrics, Medstar Georgetown University Hospital, Georgetown University Medical Center, Washington, DC

JEFF Q. BOSTIC, MD, EdD
Professor of Psychiatry, Department of Psychiatry, Division of Child and Adolescent Psychiatry, MedStar Georgetown University Hospital, Washington, DC

WILLIAM E. COPELAND, PhD
Division of Child Psychiatry, Department of Psychiatry, Vermont Center for Children, Youth, and Families, University of Vermont, Burlington, Vermont

GRACE CUSHMAN, MS
Doctoral Candidate, University of Georgia, Athens, Georgia

ELIZABETH DENTE, BA
Georgetown University School of Medicine, Washington, DC

VINAY DEVADANAM, BS
Burlington, Vermont

LAUREN DEWEY, PhD
Postdoctoral Associate, Department of Psychiatry, University of Vermont, Burlington, Vermont

R. MEREDITH ELKINS, PhD
Clinical Psychologist, McLean Anxiety Mastery Program, McLean Hospital, Belmont, Massachusetts; Instructor in Psychiatry, Harvard Medical School, Cambridge, Massachusetts

DANIEL K. HOSKER, MD
Physician, Psychiatry, Massachusetts General Hospital, Boston, Massachusetts

JIM HUDZIAK, MD
Professor, Thomas M. Achenbach Endowed Chair in Developmental Psychopathology, Departments of Psychiatry, Medicine, Pediatrics, and Communication Sciences and Disorders, Division of Child Psychiatry, Department of Psychiatry, Vermont Center for Children, Youth, and Families, University of Vermont, Burlington, Vermont

MASHA Y. IVANOVA, PhD
Assistant Professor, Departments of Psychiatry and Psychological Science, University of Vermont, Burlington, Vermont

SHASHANK V. JOSHI, MD
Director of Training in Child & Adolescent Psychiatry, Director of School Mental Health Services, Lucile Packard Children's Hospital at Stanford, Stanford, California; Associate Professor of Psychiatry, Pediatrics, and Education, Stanford University School of Medicine, Stanford, California

DAVID L. KAYE, MD
Professor of Psychiatry, Department of Psychiatry, Erie County Medical Center, Jacobs School of Medicine, University at Buffalo, Buffalo, New York

JESSICA A. KING, MA
Division of Child Psychiatry, Department Psychiatry, Vermont Center for Children, Youth, and Families, University of Vermont, Burlington, Vermont

MATTHEW LERNER, PhD
Division of Child Psychiatry, Department of Psychiatry, Vermont Center for Children, Youth, and Families, University of Vermont, Burlington, Vermont

ERIN T. MATHIS, PhD
Assistant Professor, Department of Psychiatry, Center for Child and Human Development, Georgetown University Medical Center, Washington, DC

MEGAN McCORMICK, PhD
Assistant Professor, Georgetown University, Washington, DC

KYLE H. O'BRIEN, PhD, DHSc, MSW, MSOT, LCSW, OTR/L
Assistant Professor, Department of Social Work, Southern Connecticut State University, New Haven, Connecticut

MONA P. POTTER, MD
Medical Director of McLean Hospital, Child and Adolescent Psychiatry Outpatient Services, Belmont, Massachusetts; Instructor in Psychiatry, Harvard Medical School, Cambridge, Massachusetts

SEAN PUSTILNIK, MD
Assistant Professor, Division of Child and Adolescent Psychiatry, Medstar Georgetown University Hospital, Georgetown University School of Medicine, Washington, DC

DAVID C. RETTEW, MD
Associate Professor of Psychiatry and Pediatrics, University of Vermont Larner College of Medicine, Burlington, Vermont; Medical Director, Child, Adolescent, and Family Unit, Vermont Department of Mental Health, Waterbury, Vermont; Director, Pediatric Psychiatry Clinic, University of Vermont Medical Center, Burlington, Vermont

JEFF RETTEW, PhD
Division of Child Psychiatry, Department of Psychiatry, Vermont Center for Children, Youth, and Families, University of Vermont, Burlington, Vermont

ANDREW J. ROSENFELD, MD
Assistant Professor, Psychiatry and Pediatrics, Vermont Center for Children, Youth and Families, University of Vermont Larner College of Medicine, Burlington, Vermount

ANTHONY L. ROSTAIN, MD, MA
Professor of Psychiatry and Pediatrics, Perelman School of Medicine, University of Pennsylvania, Philadelphia, Pennsylvania

ISAAC SATZ
Swarthmore College, Swarthmore, Pennsylvania

ALAN DANIEL SCHLECHTER, MD
Clinical Assistant Professor, Department of Child and Adolescent Psychiatry, NYU Langone Health, Director, Outpatient Child and Adolescent Psychiatry, Bellevue Hospital, Hassenfeld Children's Hospital at NYU Langone, Child Study Center, New York, New York

COLIN STEWART, MD
Training Director, Child and Adolescent Psychiatry, Psychiatry Clerkship Director, Assistant Clinical Professor of Psychiatry, Georgetown University Medical Center, School of Medicine, Washington, DC

PAMELA SWIFT, PhD
Assistant Professor, Department of Psychiatry, University of Vermont, Burlington, Vermont

STEVE SZOPINSKI, MS
Vice Provost, Dean of Students Office, University of Vermont, Nicholson House, Burlington, Vermont

CHRISTOPHER R. THOMAS, MD
Robert L. Stubblefield Professor of Child Psychiatry, University of Texas Medical Branch-Galveston, Galveston, Texas

STANLEY WEINBERGER, MD
Assistant Professor, Department of Pediatrics, University of Vermont, Burlington, Vermont

Contents

Well-Being Components

David C. Rettew

> Training and practice within child psychiatry has focused predominantly on mental illness rather than mental health. A growing body of evidence, however, is demonstrating the importance for clinicians also to be able to focus directly on enhancing positive traits and emotions and increasing well-being and health promotion in their patients. This complementary aspect of mental health care has been called well-being and positive psychiatry, among other terms. Being able to apply these principles to standard practice requires new knowledge, skills, and attitudes that are not part of traditional psychiatric training.

Andrew J. Rosenfeld

> Increasing behavioral data support the value of developing positive traits and attitudes to promote mental health and human flourishing. A neuroscience approach to understanding the mechanisms of the key constructs of optimism and compassion is relevant toward improving identification and measurement of relevant traits, progress and barriers to cultivating these traits, and identifying which mental health–promoting practices are most effective in promoting growth of optimism and compassion.

Megan McCormick and Grace Cushman

> This article provides a framework for understanding the application of positive psychology, in particular, Seligman's PERMA, in the context of chronic childhood illness. In particular, inflammatory bowel disease is a chronic illness that is often associated with social and emotional challenges for youth diagnosed with this lifelong condition. Specific disease factors that seemingly work against happiness are explained, and traditional notions of happiness are discussed and redefined. With PERMA as a guide, adult caregivers (eg, psychiatrists, psychologists, parents, gastroenterologists) can help youth living with chronic illness practice acceptance, adjust expectations, and find meaning, fulfillment, and psychological well-being.

Integration into Clinical Psychiatry

> In traditional medical practice, the diagnostic interview is focused on symptom collection, diagnosis, and treatment. The psychiatric interview is based on the medical model, but mental health clinicians lack the tests found in general medicine. Rapport is the most essential tool for the psychiatrist to uncover symptoms and develop a diagnosis and treatment plan. This article brings a scientific lens to the psychiatric interview. Under this microscope the value of eliciting the patient's well-being at the outset of the interview becomes clear. Using positive psychology, an evidenced-based rationale for the positive assessment is outlined and methodology and practice of the assessment reviewed.

> The medical benefits to youth conferred by physical activity, balanced nutrition, and quality sleep have been increasingly encouraged by medical and mental health providers. Emerging evidence continues to reveal benefits for youth mental health and well-being, including for youth with psychiatric disorders. This evidence seems multifactorial through both neurobiological and psychosocial systems, with common mechanisms present between physical activity, nutrition, and sleep. This article reviews the benefits of optimizing physical activity, nutrition, and sleep; how to assess these lifestyle domains with patients and their parents; and appropriate interventions to optimize well-being in youth.

> Music is a significant part of daily life for most youth, affording clinical opportunities to cultivate positive emotions, engagement, relationships, meaning, and accomplishment. Clinical inquiry into what types of music elicit different emotions, how music fits into daily life routines, how music connects one to others, and how music anchors life events can improve the clinician–patient alliance and patient well-being practices. Music may be useful in home and school settings to help youth manage diverse moods. Practicing an instrument effectively accelerates accomplishment and pleasure, which applies to other life activities.

> Mindfulness-based interventions for adults, children, and families have grown considerably, and burgeoning evidence supports use of these

approaches for a range of clinical presentations, including anxiety, depression, ADHD, and addiction. Research into the mechanisms of mindfulness suggests improvements in key brain-based functions including attentional control and emotional regulation. Mindfulness may be relevant for improving emotional and behavioral symptoms in children and families presenting for psychiatric care and also may be an important universal strategy to promote brain health. Child psychiatrists should be familiar with mindfulness-based clinical programs and also may seek to develop mindfulness-based strategies to use in clinical practice.

Traditional child psychiatry practices focus on children's symptoms and families' deficits. Focusing on goals and strengths can prepare patients and families for what they can do to enhance their health. The evidence-base for well-being practices supports integration into contemporary practice. Practical guidelines are described for using the initial assessment to address well-being practices, and to plan treatment with psychoeducation, motivational interviewing, and ongoing monitoring. Engaging and effective clinical strategies can further support and build patient and family well-being.

Emerging Topics in Well-Being

The Vermont Family Based Approach (VFBA) is an innovative approach to healthcare delivery that addresses challenges of the healthcare system in the United States. The authors conducted a randomized controlled trial of the VFBA at a primary care pediatric clinic. The goal of the trial was to test the feasibility of the VFBA in pediatrics and to improve healthcare engagement and health outcomes for families. This article presents initial results of the trial on feasibility and engagement. The VFBA was found feasible and was associated with a significant increase in engagement with health and wellness supports and services.

The University of Vermont Wellness Environment program is a neuroscience-inspired, incentive-based behavioral change program designed to improve health and academic outcomes in college-age students. The program uses health promotion and illness prevention delivered in classrooms, residential halls, and via a customized App that incentivizes healthy behaviors and monitors the use of health-promoting activities. This article presents feasibility data on participation of college students in ongoing data collection about key outcomes related to health and well-being. The data collection component were easily implemented in college students and yielded high-quality data.

Psychiatric training for medical students, residents, and fellows can integrate well-being principles to improve mental health. From preschool to college, principles of wellness and health promotion are increasingly prevalent and are showing promising results. Courses on happiness and well-being have been embraced at colleges and universities. Well-being is now a required component of child and adolescent psychiatry training. Training residents and fellows in emotional and behavioral well-being requires incorporation into clinical supervision and the overall culture and infrastructure of the training program.

Child psychiatrists should play an active role in helping parents and children to develop healthy media use habits and can introduce uses of technology including mobile applications and telepsychiatry to enhance clinical care. Strength-based approaches in clinical assessment and treatment build patient and family engagement and enhance outcomes in child psychiatry. Focusing on supporting youths' strengths and enhancing emotional and behavioral well-being are critical strategies for child psychiatrists working in consultation with schools and other community settings, and in advocating for optimal environments for children and families.

CHILD AND ADOLESCENT PSYCHIATRIC CLINICS

SERIES OF RELATED INTEREST

Psychiatric Clinics of North America
Pediatric Clinics of North America
Neurologic Clinics

AACAP Members: Please go to www.jaacap.org for information on access to the Child and Adolescent Psychiatric Clinics. *Resident* Members of AACAP: Special access information is available at www.childpsych.theclinics.com.

THE CLINICS ARE AVAILABLE ONLINE!
Access your subscription at:
www.theclinics.com

Preface

The Science of Well-Being: Integration into Clinical Child Psychiatry

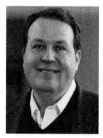   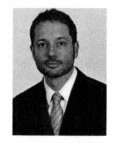   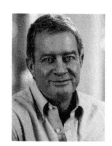

David C. Rettew, MD   Matthew G. Biel, MD, MSc   Jeff Q. Bostic, MD, EdD
Editors

Most child psychiatrists and other mental health professions want patients not only to get better but also to be *well*. Relieving people of symptoms like intense sadness and anxiety is undoubtedly an important goal, but are our traditional tools of psychotherapy and medication enough to bring people sufficient relief to move them toward states of happiness, fulfillment, and productivity? For many mental health professionals, it has seemed our goals have been too modest, and our toolbox too small. Fortunately, a growing literature about the science of emotional-behavioral well-being can now inform clinicians interested and willing to expand their focus and expertise. This issue of *Child and Adolescent Psychiatric Clinics of North America* distills key information from this growing evidence base and offers practical guidelines and suggestions to help clinicians incorporate these advances into day-to-day practice.

The issue is divided into three sections. The first, *Well-Being Components*, introduces the concept of well-being into a child psychiatry context with some important background information describing the history, controversies, and advances that have brought us to this point. Also included in this section are articles devoted to the neuroscience of well-being, and the components of well-being that can be applied in treating individuals suffering from chronic illness. The second section, *Integration into Clinical Psychiatry*, provides rich discussion of the evidence base supporting the clinical applications of mindfulness, exercise, sleep, and good nutrition in child psychiatry. These components help to build and nourish healthy brain development and are exquisitely applicable components of a comprehensive treatment plan for youth struggling with mental health challenges. The articles in these sections go beyond summarizing the science by also offering recommendations as to how mental health clinicians can assess these dimensions during evaluations and include them in regular follow-up

Child Adolesc Psychiatric Clin N Am 28 (2019) xiii–xiv
https://doi.org/10.1016/j.chc.2019.01.001
1056-4993/19/© 2019 Elsevier Inc. All rights reserved.

visits. Finally, the third section of the issue, *Emerging Topics in Well-Being*, explores applications of this science to primary care settings and college campuses. The final two articles deal with the education of well-being to students of all types, and aspects of well-being practice and research that are in need of further attention and refinement.

As editors, we are delighted to present this information to you and are extremely grateful to the authors for each article in this unique *Child and Adolescent Psychiatric Clinics of North America* issue applying well-being to child psychiatry practice. Our goal is not only to inform readers but also to challenge them to think about how mental health professionals should define themselves and the boundaries of their expertise and practice. We hope that most readers will find the recommendations in this issue useful for many patients and will embrace well-being as a fundamental component of their clinical mission. Cultivating comprehensive well-being in our patients is a natural (and perhaps overdue) extension of our purpose as child psychiatrists. We warmly invite you to explore this issue as we consider what it truly means to be a mental *health* professional.

David C. Rettew, MD
Child, Adolescent, and Family Division
VT Dept of Mental Health, Department of Psychiatry
University of Vermont Larner College of Medicine
1 South Prospect Street
Burlington, VT 05401, USA

Matthew G. Biel, MD, MSc
Child and Adolescent Psychiatry
MedStar Georgetown University Hospital
Georgetown University School of Medicine
2115 Wisconsin Avenue Northwest, Suite 200
Washington, DC 20007, USA

Jeff Q. Bostic, MD, EdD
Child and Adolescent Psychiatry
MedStar Georgetown University Hospital
2115 Wisconsin Avenue Northwest, Suite 200
Washington, DC 20007, USA

E-mail addresses:
david.rettew@med.uvm.edu (D.C. Rettew)
MGB101@gunet.georgetown.edu (M.G. Biel)
jbostic57@gmail.com (J.Q. Bostic)

Well-Being Components

Better than Better
The New Focus on Well-Being in Child Psychiatry

David C. Rettew, MD[a,b,c],*

KEYWORDS

- Positive psychiatry • Psychiatric training • Vermont Family-Based Approach
- Positive psychology • Well-being • Wellness

KEY POINTS

- The field of child psychiatry has historically focused more on mental illness than the positive aspects of mental functioning and how to achieve them.
- An emphasis on mental illness has ironically limited psychiatry's ability to help patients realize and address their full potential when it comes to emotional-behavioral health.
- There are good and increasing scientific data to support wellness and health promotion activities, such as physical activity, diet, mindfulness, and other behaviors, as evidence-based treatments for child psychiatric disorders.
- Models such as the Vermont Family-Based Approach have been developed to help clinicians more fully incorporate family well-being and health promotion into the delivery of child psychiatric care.
- Significant debates and gaps in knowledge persist related to many aspects of well-being and positive psychiatry.

Child psychiatrists are physicians, but they also frequently label themselves as mental health professionals. The words "mental" and "professionals" certainly seem apt, but what about "health?" In thinking more closely about the way child psychiatrists are trained and deployed, one might quite easily come to the conclusion that a more accurate term for them might be mental *illness* professionals.[1] They learn about depression, but rarely happiness. They try to prevent adverse child experiences, but can stumble in suggesting what should take their place. They get involved when people are struggling, but often see their job as being completed once a patient is feeling "better." Open the Web page on "mental health information" from the National Institute of Mental *Health*, and what one sees is a list of psychiatric *disorders*.[2] Indeed,

Disclosure Statement: No financials relationships to disclose.
[a] University of Vermont Larner College of Medicine, Burlington, VT, USA; [b] Child, Adolescent, and Family Unit, Vermont Department of Mental Health, Waterbury, VT, USA; [c] Pediatric Psychiatry Clinic, University of Vermont Medical Center, 1 South Prospect Street, Arnold 3, Burlington, VT 05401, USA
* 1 South Prospect Street, Arnold 3, Burlington, VT 05401.
E-mail address: David.rettew@med.uvm.edu

Child Adolesc Psychiatric Clin N Am 28 (2019) 127–135
https://doi.org/10.1016/j.chc.2018.11.001
1056-4993/19/© 2018 Elsevier Inc. All rights reserved.

American Academy of Child and Adolescent Psychiatry defines the profession as "a physician who specializes in the diagnosis and the treatment of disorders of thinking, feeling and/or behavior affecting children, adolescents, and their families."[3] This explanation certainly seems to accurately reflect education and practice but, lately, people are beginning to ask the question of *should it*? Happiness, after all, is hardly the simple absence of depression, and the ability to focus and concentrate can certainly go beyond the mere absence of an attention "deficit." As stated by Seligman and Csikszentmihalyi,[4(pp6)] "Raising children, I realized, is vastly more than fixing what is wrong with them. It is about identifying and nurturing their strongest qualities, what they own and are best at, and helping them find niches in which they can best live out these strengths."

This issue of *Child and Adolescent Psychiatry Clinics of North America* examines the case for psychiatrists and other mental health professionals to expand their expertise and clinical attention beyond the domain of symptom reduction and into the realm of true well-being. It looks at the evidence and neuroscience behind health-promoting behaviors, such as exercise, sleep, mindfulness, music participation, positive parenting, and other activities as brain building techniques that are deserving of clinical attention, not only for youth who are already progressing typically but also for those who are struggling with psychopathology. Unfortunately, cultural pressures in many western societies work against youth being able to engage in wellness endeavors, such as music and regular exercise, especially in the transition from midchildhood into adolescence. As children age, the opportunities to participate on sports teams and musical activities often fade for those lacking high levels of innate skill,[5] leaving many who could derive much benefit from these activities without good access. Financial constraints and busy parent schedules can also conspire to limit opportunities for youth to participate in behaviors that promote optimal brain development. As these realities confront research demonstrating that wellness activities may provide the most benefit from those who possess the least intrinsic talent for them,[6] a compelling argument begins to be made for child psychiatrists and other clinicians to focus more actively on these domains.

Thus, for many clinicians, the issue is no longer *if* they should incorporate more wellness and health promotion into their daily practice but *how*. Psychiatrists traditionally have found themselves in the role of the individual therapist, the psychopharmacologist, or both, spending a large percentage of their time on what might be called the "Three Ss" of scars, symptoms, and side effects. Now, however, there is the opportunity to incorporate findings from an increasingly robust literature demonstrating that the ability to expand the focus beyond the child to the whole family, and from illness to well-being, provides a more comprehensive toolbox from which one can help patients overcome difficulties and thrive. The articles in this issue provide a roadmap to help child psychiatrists identify and emphasize a child and family's strengths during treatment, cultivate the development of positive emotions and skills, and integrate more fully family-based well-being and health promotion behaviors. These articles can help clinicians apply the science in several wellness domains and initiatives to everyday practice. Admittedly, the psychiatrist who wishes to integrate these principles in their routine care may initially find it challenging to do so within the contemporary "med check" model of treatment. However, more family-oriented, well-being focused care can be readily adapted into one's standard routines without the need for radical transformation, especially for psychiatrists who already work collaboratively with other types of mental health professionals. Indeed, such a direction reflects the tradition as child psychiatrists of prioritizing a child's optimal growth and development within larger systems of care.

A BRIEF HISTORICAL CONTEXT

One could argue that, up until relatively recently, the entire field of child psychiatry has evolved by slowly expanding its "jurisdiction" from more narrowly focused areas, such as a child's fantasy life, to ever broader spheres that encompass not only the individual child but also his or her entire environment, including parents, the school, and peers. Broadening from a more disease-oriented approach toward a greater appreciation of the need to consider the positive elements of mental health dates back to William James and his beliefs in the healing properties of positive thoughts and emotions.[7] A resurgence in this perspective occurred with the advent of the humanistic psychology tradition and pioneers such as Abraham Maslow[8] and the appreciation of a hierarchy of needs, and Carl Rogers with his concentration on self-esteem.[9] Even before the dawn of modern psychiatry, the importance of human virtues was noted by ancient Greek philosophers such as Aristotle,[10] whereas wellness practices such as mindfulness have been with us for thousands of years.

Jumping forward to the 1990s, psychologist Martin Seligman, initially known for work on the phenomenon of learned helplessness, turned his focus toward human strengths, virtues, and well-being. As president of the American Psychological Association, Seligman successfully advocated that psychologists devote significant research attention to the field of "positive psychology" to better understand subjective states, such as well-being and contentment, individual traits such as hope and optimism, and thriving communities that foster qualities like responsibility and altruism.[4] This call to action inspired the revival of positive psychology as a legitimate target of scientific inquiry and a genuine movement began on an international scale that continues to this day.

One might wonder how the field of psychiatry reacted to this shift. Certainly, many psychiatrists had for years been concerned with what underlies optimal human development, including George Valliant and the Harvard Study of Adult Development,[11] Irvin Yalom and existential psychotherapy,[12] C. Robert Cloninger and the science of well-being,[13] and many involved in the recovery movement.[10,14] However, psychiatry was also engaged with the "decade of the brain" during the 1990s and the potential promises of new pharmacologic treatments for struggling youth. These developments, coupled with the training as physicians dedicated first and foremost to helping those who are ill, may have understandably delayed the collective attention to well-being. In Seligman's 1998 presidential address to the American Psychological Association, he notes that focus on the positive aspects of mental health waned as psychologists increasing saw themselves as a "healing profession" rather than a discipline devoted to improving the lives of all.[15] Ironically, however, increasing clinical and neuroscience research now suggests that a "wellness orientation versus medical model" approach is a false dichotomy, because many health promotion behaviors show great promise not only as preventative measures but also as frequently missed opportunities for treatment.

The term "positive psychiatry" was proposed by geriatric psychiatrist Dilip Jeste, while President of the American Psychiatric Association in 2012. Jeste's focus was inspired by research that demonstrated a somewhat surprising trend related to increasing levels of happiness and contentment in the process of aging, even as many signs of objective health were beginning to wane.[16] These observations led to more global efforts to highlight the importance of positive psychiatry as an underdeveloped component of the field.[15]

With its emphasis on a developmental perspective and attention to the growth-promoting or -restricting qualities of an individual's environment, child psychiatry would seem like an especially good home for those interested in well-being and the principles of positive psychiatry. However, here too a disease and symptom-based model has predominated, in part shaped by changes in health care delivery and economics.[17] There have, however, been some notable exceptions, moving forward often under different terminology. One such effort that will be described in more detail in subsequent articles of this issue is the Vermont Family-Based Approach (VFBA), which was developed by child psychiatrist Jim Hudziak.[18] This model describes a mental health care delivery system applicable not only to child psychiatric treatment clinics but also in preventive contexts within primary care and public health. Using collaborative efforts from family wellness coaches, psychotherapists, and family-based psychiatrists, the VFBA aims to optimize family functioning and incorporate several wellness and health promotion activities (such as physical exercise, music, good nutrition, mindfulness) into a family's daily structure. It also directly tries to maximize the positive influence of parents through the use of evidence-based parent behavioral training and formal mental health screening and treatment of parental psychopathology. This training is delivered not from the perspective that parents are necessarily *deficient* in their skills but from research demonstrating that more behaviorally challenging children are particularly sensitive to both the negative and the positive aspects of parenting behavior.[19]

Others in child psychiatry have similarly converged on the idea that both rapport and treatment outcomes with patients can be enhanced when clinicians spend some time focusing on what's *right* with patients and how to build upon positive thoughts and emotions.[20] The expanding evidence base for many wellness domains, such as nutrition, exercise, and mindfulness, has also not gone unnoticed within the field.[21–23] The end result is new avenues for intervention and a bigger toolbox for clinicians willing to learn and apply this advancing science to their practice.

WHAT IS WELL-BEING AND POSITIVE CHILD PSYCHIATRY?

For many people, the term "wellness" or "well-being" conjures images of beautiful people already functioning at a high level, with extra time and energy on their hands, practicing yoga on a beach as the sun rises slowly above the ocean. With this stereotype in mind, it is easy to dismiss the practice of wellness and the science of well-being as distractions that can take a psychiatrist away from the critical work required to alleviate the suffering of people grappling with acute and chronic mental illness.

The reality, however, is much less ethereal and far more relevant. At the same time, it is also true that researchers and advocates of the "other" side of mental health have used different terminology to describe partially overlapping constructs, and these applications can be confusing to newcomers in this area. Some of these terms still have yet to be completely defined and delineated from related concepts. As a primer for some of the vocabulary that will be encountered in subsequent articles, a short description of some of the key concepts and terminology in these evolving areas may be useful.

Well-Being

There remains no official consensus over the precise definition of well-being, although attempts have been made to use the term to describe more than just the hedonic state of feeling happy so to include other components of positive functioning.[24] Seligman has advanced a popular model that defines well-being as the presence of positive emotions, engagement, (positive) relationships, meaning, and accomplishment under the acronym *PERMA*.[25]

Positive Psychology

Positive psychology has been defined as "the scientific study of what makes life worth living."[26] It describes a field that seeks to understand human strengths and virtues and the elements that enable individuals and communities to function at their best. It also strives to develop techniques that enable people to achieve their maximum well-being. As described above, the term developed from the work of Seligman and his colleagues in the 1990s, although was never intended to be in the exclusive realm of psychologists.

Positive Psychiatry

Following in the footsteps of positive psychology, the field of positive psychiatry has been described as, "the science and practice of psychiatry that seeks to understand and promote well-being through assessments and interventions aimed at enhancing positive psychosocial factors among people who have or are at high risk for developing mental and physical illnesses."[10] Although there is clearly enough overlap between the two constructs to inspire hope for there to eventually be an umbrella label for both, this definition suggests perhaps a closer affinity to the field of medicine and an increased emphasis on work with individuals who are challenged with mental health problems. Both positive psychology and positive psychiatry take pains to articulate that these extensions are meant not to replace but to complement a more traditional focus on mental health disorders.

Positive Psychotherapy

Specific techniques that are used to enhance positive emotions and traits and that exist at least somewhat independently from more traditional counseling and psychotherapy practices are often referred to as positive psychotherapy or positive psychology interventions. To be sure, the tenets of positive psychology or psychiatry are already subsumed in many types of psychotherapy.[27] However, these techniques are built specifically to enhance positive emotions and other PERMA components.[28] An example of one of the most well-known techniques is the gratitude exercise in which someone writes a list or even a letter of gratitude to someone who has helped them in the past. These techniques can be done with people who do or do not meet criteria for a psychiatric disorder.

The Vermont Family-Based Approach

As described above, the VFBA is a specific clinical model that was developed by Hudziak at the University of Vermont.[18,29] Although certainly consistent with many aspects described as positive psychiatry, the model was designed specifically for families and places much emphasis on parenting behavior and parental mental health. Wellness activities, such as mindfulness, musical training, and exercise, are "prescribed" for all members of the family, and the model is applicable for those without existing psychopathology. The VFBA and its implementation in the primary care setting are described later in this issue.

CHALLENGES TO THE WELL-BEING APPROACH

Well-being and methods to cultivate it have become an important topic over the past three decades in both lay and professional circles. With that popularity, however, has emerged some criticism and concern. Although efforts to incorporate emotional-behavioral wellness more fully into the scope of psychiatry seem like a natural, even obvious, direction in which psychiatry should move, it is not without detractors.[30]

Some are concerned that an increased focus on well-being will take away much needed resources from more severely affected individuals. Others see an emphasis on wellness as a potential empathic failure, because clinicians attempt to dismiss very real suffering and trauma with "happy thoughts." The evidence-based and scientific validity of some wellness-related interventions has also been challenged.

Many of these concerns are well founded, highlighting legitimate complexities within this emerging discipline. It is certainly true that recent years have witnessed the explosion of several trends making grandiose claims of their efficacy in the absence of good scientific data.[31] From body cleansing "detox" procedures to "crystal healing," many of these claims come with specific products to buy, books to read, and clinicians to see. Sadly, an unfortunate byproduct of the important effort to repudiate the vast amount of misinformation pervading the public is that more legitimate and scientifically supported health promotion activities, such as mindfulness, can get lumped into the same pseudoscience basket. That said, it will remain important for researchers of well-being and advocates of positive psychiatry not to let the level of enthusiasm move ahead of the available data.

In the author's view, perhaps the biggest misunderstanding underlying the pursuit of well-being is that these endeavors help only those people who are already healthy. The research, however, clearly speaks otherwise in demonstrating the benefits of wellness and health promotion for those challenged by existing psychopathology or at significant risk of developing clinically significant behavioral problems. For example, the Harmony Project (https://www.harmony-project.org) is a musical training and mentorship program that originated in Los Angeles to help disadvantaged youth. At first glance, it is easy to think that children growing up with poverty, violence, and economic disadvantage have much bigger problems than not knowing how to play a violin. However, the data show that their participation in the program can counteract some of the negative effects of their adversity.[32] In addition to the direct neurodevelopmental benefits of playing an instrument, these children also benefit from being part of structured community while building skills and a sense of accomplishment that help them graduate and succeed in college and beyond.[33]

Other well-being activities have also shown value among youth with a wide range of emotional-behavioral problems and diagnoses. Exercise, for example, has been shown to be beneficial in those with attention-deficit/hyperactivity disorder,[34] while mindfulness-based practices show promise for anxiety and other symptoms.[35–37] Indeed, it is provocative but probably quite fair at this point to state that the magnitude of the evidence for many wellness interventions now exceeds that for many pediatric off-label uses of medications that have found their way to common practice. More and more, a direct focus on well-being within the world of child psychiatry can no longer be considered "fringe" or "alternate."

A lingering debate has been whether illness and well-being are best considered to lie along a single continuum versus being two distinct but mutually overlapping dimensions. There are increasing data now to suggest the latter.[27] Although considerable evidence now suggests that psychopathology is itself dimensional,[38] these continuums appear to exist at least somewhat independently from positive qualities and attributes, with both shared and distinct correlates with other family and environmental factors.[39] These studies correspond with what many mental health professionals observe clinically, namely, that some patients with diagnosable conditions are also endowed with many positive qualities that can serve them well in overcoming their symptoms, whereas for others these traits require more cultivation and practice.

It is also a myth of positive psychiatry that its goal is to create some kind of Pollyanna state that ignores human suffering and evades more difficult, yet necessary conversations. Psychiatrists will always be committed to individuals struggling with severe and chronic psychiatric illness. Indeed, one of the primary lessons from the recovery movement was the importance of not only alleviating symptoms but also assisting people to find meaning in their lives as they reestablish important social roles and relationships.[14] Clinicians who can find ways to guide and inspire individuals toward improved well-being similarly acknowledge that patients are more than their "bag of symptoms"[40] with aspirations for connection, purpose, and achievement just like everyone else. Achieving this, however, requires a set of knowledge, skills, and attitudes beyond what most of us obtained during psychiatric training.

SUMMARY

Although the field of child psychiatry has always kept the idea of well-being and health promotion in its peripheral vision, it has struggled to look it directly in the eye. This shortcoming, however, is now changing as accumulating research demonstrates the value of enhancing positive emotions and well-being for children and families regardless of whether they are already functioning at a high level or grappling with serious emotional-behavioral problems. This emphasis, which has been called positive psychiatry by some, is designed as a complement, rather than as a replacement, to the more traditional disease-based approach that receives the most attention in current psychiatric training and practice. Real-world methods and techniques are also being developed to allow child psychiatrists and other clinicians the ability to incorporate these advances into their day-to-day care with patients. Revising the mission of child psychiatry to include the entire spectrum of mental functioning is an exciting development, even if it requires acquiring new knowledge, skills, and health care approaches. This issue of *Child and Adolescent Psychiatry Clinics of North America* on the science of well-being is a valuable resource for those looking to develop their expertise as true mental *health* professionals.

REFERENCES

1. Rettew DC. Child psychiatrists should be mental HEALTH professionals. JAACAP Connect 2018;5:6–9.
2. National Institute of Mental Health. Mental health information. Available at: https://www.nimh.nih.gov/health/topics/index.shtml. Accessed July 25, 2018.
3. America Academy of Child & Adolescent Psychiatry. What is child and adolescent psychiatry? Available at: https://dev.aacap.org/AACAP/Medical_Students_and_Residents/Medical_Students/What_is_Child_and_Adolescent_Psychiatry.aspx. Accessed July 25, 2018.
4. Seligman MEP, Csikszentmihalyi M. Positive psychology: an introduction. Am Psychol 2000;55:5–14.
5. Huppertz C, Bartels M, Van Beijsterveldt CE, et al. Effect of shared environmental factors on exercise behavior from age 7 to 12 years. Med Sci Sports Exerc 2012;44:2025–32.
6. Grape C, Sandgren M, Hansson LO, et al. Does singing promote well-being?: an empirical study of professional and amateur singers during a singing lesson. Integr Physiol Behav Sci 2003;38:65–74.
7. Froh JJ. The history of positive psychology: truth be told. N Y State Psychol 2004;16:18–20.
8. Maslow A. Toward a psychology of being. New York: Simon & Schuster; 1962.
9. Rogers C. On becoming a person: a therapist's view of psychotherapy. New York: Houghton Mifflin Company; 1961.

10. Boxorgnia B, Summers RF, Jeste DV. Overview of positive psychiatry. In: Summers RF, Jeste DV, editors. Positive psychiatry: a casebook. Washington (DC): American Psychiatric Association Press; 2018. p. 1–26.
11. Vaillant GE. Aging well: surprising guideposts to a happier life from the Landmark Study of Adult Development. New York: Little, Brown; 2008.
12. Yalom ID. Existential psychotherapy. New York: Basic Books; 1980.
13. Cloninger CR. Feeling good: the science of well-being. Oxford (England): Oxford University Press; 2004.
14. Slade M. Mental illness and well-being: the central importance of positive psychology and recovery approaches. BMC Health Serv Res 2010;10:26.
15. Jeste DV, Palmer BW. Introduction: what is positive psychiatry. In: Jeste DV, Palmer BW, editors. Positive psychiatry: a clinical handbook. Washington (DC): American Psychiatric Publishing; 2015.
16. Jeste DV, Savla GN, Thompson WK, et al. Association between older age and more successful aging: critical role of resilience and depression. Am J Psychiatry 2013;170:188–96.
17. Jeste DV, Palmer BW, Rettew DC, et al. Positive psychiary: its time has come. J Clin Psychiatry 2015;76:675–83.
18. Hudziak J, Ivanova MY. The Vermont family based approach: family based health promotion, illness prevention, and intervention. Child Adolesc Psychiatr Clin N Am 2016;25:167–78.
19. Slagt M, Dubas JS, Dekovic M, et al. Differences in sensitivity to parenting depending on child temperament: a meta-analysis. Psychol Bull 2016;142:1068–110.
20. O'Brien KH, Schlechter A. Is talking about what's wrong necessarily right: a positive perspective on the diagnostic interview. J Am Acad Child Adolesc Psychiatry 2016;55:262–4.
21. Simkin DR, Black NB. Meditation and mindfulness in clinical practice. Child Adolesc Psychiatr Clin N Am 2014;23:487–534.
22. Brown HE, Pearson N, Braithwaite RE, et al. Physical activity interventions and depression in children and adolescents: a systematic review and meta-analysis. Sports Med 2013;43:195–206.
23. Bloch MH, Qawasmi A. Omega-3 fatty acid supplementation for the treatment of children with attention-deficit/hyperactivity disorder symptomatology: systematic review and meta-analysis. J Am Acad Child Adolesc Psychiatry 2011;50:991–1000.
24. Schultze-Lutter F, Schimmelmann BG, Schmidt SJ. Resilience, risk, mental health and well-being: associations and conceptual differences. Eur Child Adolesc Psychiatry 2016;25:459–66.
25. Seligman MEP. Flourish: a visionary new understanding of happiness and well-being. New York: Free Press; 2011.
26. Peterson C. What Is positive psychology and what is it not? Psychol Today Blog 2008. Available at: https://www.psychologytoday.com/us/blog/the-good-life/200805/what-is-positive-psychology-and-what-is-it-not. Accessed October 1, 2018.
27. Summers RF, Lord JA. Positivity in supportive and psychodynamic therapy. In: Jeste DV, Palmer BW, editors. Positive psychiatry: a clinical handbook. Washington (DC): American Psychiatric Publishing; 2015. p. 167–92.
28. Seligman MEP. Positive psychotherapy. Am Psychol 2006;61:774–88.
29. Hudziak JJ. Genetic and environmental influences on wellness, resilience, and psychopathology: a family-based approach for promotion, prevention, and

intervention. In: Hudziak JJ, editor. Developmental psychopathology and well-ness: genetic and environmental influences. Washington (DC): American Psychiatric Publishing, Inc; 2008. p. 267–86.

30. Held BS. The negative side of positive psychology. J Humanistic Psychol 2004; 44:9–46.
31. Lilienfeld SO. Introduction to special section on pseudoscience in psychiatry. Can J Psychiatry 2015;60:531–3.
32. Kraus N, Hornickel J, Strait DL, et al. Engagement in community music classes sparks neuroplasticity and language development in children from disadvantaged backgrounds. Front Psychol 2014;5:1403.
33. Harmony project - our impact. 2018. Available at: https://www.harmonyprojectofamerica. org/-by-the-numbers.html. Accessed August 21, 2018.
34. Vysniauske R, Verburgh L, Oosterlaan J, et al. The effects of physical exercise on functional outcomes in the treatment of ADHD: a meta-analysis. J Atten Disord 2016. [Epub ahead of print].
35. Biegel GM, Brown KW, Shapiro SL, et al. Mindfulness-based stress reduction for the treatment of adolescent psychiatric outpatients: a randomized clinical trial. J Consult Clin Psychol 2009;77:855–66.
36. Zoogman S, Goldberg SB, Hoyt WT, et al. Mindfulness interventions with youth: a meta-analysis. Mindfulness 2015;6:290–302.
37. Fulweiler B, John RM. Mind & body practices in the treatment of adolescent anxiety. Nurse Pract 2018;43:36–43.
38. Rettew DC. Child temperament: new thinking about the boundary between traits and illness. New York: W.W. Norton & Company; 2013.
39. Patalay P, Fitzsimons E. Correlates of mental illness and wellbeing in children: are they the same? results from the UK Millennium Cohort Study. J Am Acad Child Adolesc Psychiatry 2016;55:771–83.
40. Hoffman E. The right to be human: a biography of Abraham Maslow. New York: St. Martin's Press; 1988.

The Neuroscience of Happiness and Well-Being
What Brain Findings from Optimism and Compassion Reveal

Andrew J. Rosenfeld, MD

KEYWORDS

- Optimism • Compassion • Well-being • Neuroscience

KEY POINTS

- Adding a focus on cultivating well-being recognizes the disparity between a lack of diagnosable mental illness versus the presence of human flourishing.
- Work done to understand the brain's role in generating and maintaining psychological and physical well-being is in its infancy, yet has identified some consistent structures and networks implicated in positive characteristics, such as optimism and compassion.
- Traits like compassion and optimism show consistent behavioral and health benefits that contribute to well-being.
- The neuroscience of well-being holds promise in determining which practices build neural networks subserving positive traits and mindsets that can promote mental health, prevent mental illness, and reduce or offset symptom burden.

Folks are usually about as happy as they make up their minds to be.
—Attributed to Abraham Lincoln[1]

The value of viewing psychiatry as "clinical neuroscience,"[2] aligns with the stated Accreditation Council for Graduate Medical Education goals through the Child and Adolescent Psychiatry Milestone Project.[3] The Milestones reference the psychiatrist's mastery of neurobiology and applied neuroscience to "integrat[e] knowledge of neurobiology into advocacy for psychiatric patient care and stigma reduction," understand neurodevelopment, and optimize case formulation and treatment planning.[3] An understanding of neuroscientific concepts is thus relevant to day-to-day psychiatric work as well as the future practice of the specialty.

And although pediatric psychiatry has represented itself publicly as devoted to the treatment of mental illnesses,[4] this issue of the *Child and Adolescent Psychiatric*

Disclosure Statement: None applicable.
Psychiatry and Pediatrics, Vermont Center for Children, Youth and Families, University of Vermont Larner College of Medicine, 1 South Prospect Street, Burlington, VT 05401, USA
E-mail address: Andrew.rosenfeld@uvmhealth.org

Clinics of North America balances prevention and wellness promotion in our patients with the assessment and treatment of psychopathology. Clinical approaches to promote well-being are grounded in behavioral strategies and are increasingly supported by neuroscientific evidence describing the brain-based impacts of these strategies. Pairing perspectives from neuroscience and clinical experience promises to create and optimize health promotion efforts and to support our efforts to educate the public and our patients about the human mind.

As the scientific study of positive psychology and psychiatry is relatively young,[5–8] the investigation of neuroscientific underpinnings for positive psychiatric concepts is understandably in early days. The landscape is changing with emerging neuroimaging technologies and data analysis tools. Although the depth and breadth of wellness evidence is growing, this article focuses on several representative areas that demonstrate the direction of the field, its challenges, and its promise.

MEASURES OF WELL-BEING

Defining and measuring happiness itself remains a considerable obstacle.[9] The variety of instruments assessing happiness suggests that there may instead be "happinesses," a heterogeneity of "flourishing" suggested by Seligman and colleagues[10] in labeling "the pleasant life, the good life, and the meaningful life" as separable entities. One approach is to evaluate specific components thought to influence current or future happiness, such as optimism, gratitude, or positive relationships.[11–13] The next wave of assessment tools is likely to include biosensors that may evaluate physiologic parameters reflecting autonomic balance, electrophysiologic activity, and/or emotional tone via facial recognition software. Combining these with behavioral and geographic tracking may convey powerful data to suggest personalized behavior change programs to improve well-being. This article addresses definitions, measurements, and techniques, in addition to reviewing results of recent investigations and tentative conclusions based on this body of work. Most of the literature focuses on adult participants, but studies of youth are expanding.

Optimism

Definitions and measurement

Optimism is most commonly defined in 2 related ways. As a *dispositional trait*, optimism refers to "people who expect good things to happen . . . [and] tend to be confident and persistent in the face of challenge."[14] The most standard measure of dispositional optimism is the Life Orientation Test–Revised (LOT-R). The LOT-R measures generalized expectancies regarding the anticipation of positive or negative life events and provides a continuous distribution of scores.

The second approach to optimism is referred to as optimistic *explanatory style*. This covers how an individual responds cognitively in the face of positive or negative events in life. For example, the pessimistic attributional style posits that a negative life event indicates a likelihood of ongoing, generalized misfortune for the foreseeable future, whereas an optimistic attributional style interprets the same event as time-limited and situation-specific. This is typically measured via the Attributional Style Questionnaire,[11] which assesses respondents' explanations of hypothetical events on the axes of permanence, pervasiveness, and personalization.

Connection to mental health

The relevance of optimism to well-being has been demonstrated consistently in several domains. For women in the postpartum period, third trimester optimism predicts lower depression ratings postpartum. For coronary artery bypass recipients, optimism correlates with less presurgical distress and greater postsurgical life satisfaction lasting up to 5 years postoperatively. Similar results can be found with various cancers, in vitro fertilization, caregiver depression and physical health, and for reduced distress and greater social connection in matriculating college students across the first semester.[14] More optimistic participants show more active, problem-focused, and positive coping styles with less denial or avoidance of problematic situations. Optimists enjoy greater physical well-being, such as less atherosclerotic development over time, less human immunodeficiency virus disease progression, faster healing responses, stronger immune responses to vaccination, and reduced all-cause mortality.[14,15]

Optimistic patients are more engaged in their health and seek more information about health conditions,[16] choose more health-promoting behaviors,[17] and avoid risky health behaviors.[18] When it comes to predicting life satisfaction and subjective well-being, optimism consistently rates as an important variable[19,20]

Neuroscience in healthy participants

Neural structures and networks surrounding optimism are being delineated using various methods. Alessandri and Pascalis[21] have used studied measures of general optimism (GO) using electroencephalography, finding evidence of higher activation of the right posterior cingulate cortex (PCC) specific to GO, whereas self-enhancing optimism correlated with activity in the left inferior frontal gyrus (IFG). These areas are often associated with self-referential thinking and cognitive control, respectively.

Along related lines, Sharot and colleagues[22,23] conducted several studies focused on the mechanisms of the optimism bias, a tendency to have unrealistically positive expectations for the future. This was connected to a decrease in the error-correction signal from the right IFG. The decreased IFG response to error was more marked in those with higher *trait* optimism. Regions including the medial frontal cortex and left IFG were implicated in updating beliefs with positive information. Kuzmanovic and colleagues[24] replicated the optimism bias but found that activity in the subgenual ventromedial prefrontal cortex (vmPFC) increased when participants used new information in a biased way to either bolster positive beliefs or minimize negative beliefs about the future. Furthermore, activity in elements of the brain's reward network, including the ventral striatum and dorsomedial prefrontal cortex (dmPFC), predicted a greater optimistic updating bias. Blair and colleagues[25] used functional magnetic resonance imaging (fMRI) to show that vmPFC and PCC activity increased with expected positive future outcomes and correlated with fewer depressive symptoms reported. Yet the rostral anterior cingulate cortex was more specifically predictive of optimistic updating based on *positive* information, and dmPFC activity was upregulated in kind with optimistic updating based on *negative* information. Dolcos and colleagues[26] showed that increased optimism mediated the link between greater orbitofrontal cortex (OFC) gray matter volume and reduced anxiety. Such work gives hope that the anatomy of optimism may present us with means to build resilience to anxiety.

Pessimism with regard to self-evaluation is in some ways definitional for depressive symptoms (eg, worthlessness, hopelessness). Wu and colleagues[27] found lower activity and connectivity of OFC and dorsolateral prefrontal cortices (dlPFC) correlated with higher standardized depression symptom ratings, whereas greater activity in the dmPFC and dlPFC synchronized with optimism measures.

Neuroscience in identified patients

Understanding optimism also may shed light on some psychopathologic conditions. Using fMRI, Blair and colleagues[28] found that those with generalized anxiety did not see positive events as likely to happen to them, and this was underpinned by functional differences in mPFC and caudate. This may represent an inability to connect self-referential thinking and reward to future positive events. Moreover, low-impact events caused greater mPFC responses in patients with generalized anxiety, possibly reflecting out-of-proportion anxious self-referential thinking.

Garrett and colleagues[29] extended these findings to those with clinical depression. Depressed participants showed more neural activity in the right IFG and the right inferior parietal lobule when updating their beliefs about the future to be more negative. More optimistic, nondepressed participants showed relatively diminished responses in these same areas.

Interventions to improve optimism

Interventions to build optimism are already showing promise in the clinical arena, from cognitive therapy,[30] to cognitive behavioral therapy,[31] to prevention programs geared at adolescents.[32,33] For example, a prevention program in primary care clinics with adolescents showed improvements in explanatory style, along with reductions in anxiety and depressive symptoms, particularly among girls and those with high symptoms initially. Outcomes improved when there was greater treatment attendance and therapist fidelity.[33] In adults with depressive disorders, explanatory style improvements were significant after a cognitive therapy and correlated with symptom improvements over time.[30]

Summary/implications

In all, the evidence for the behavioral benefits of dispositional optimism and an optimistic explanatory style are multifold and already to some extent incorporated in parts of standard psychotherapeutic interventions. Neuroscience now provides support for optimism, with growing anatomic consistency involving at least vmPFC, dmPFC, IFG, cingulate cortex, and OFC. Potentially significant gains could be achieved by furthering our understanding of the subcomponents of the construct of optimism, their utility in building flourishing mental health, and their limitations.

Compassion

Definitions and measurement

Compassion, the concern for others' welfare, encompasses 3 elements. Compassion results from bearing witness to suffering in others:

1. That is of a serious nature
2. That is the result of an unjust fate, not self-imposed
3. For which the witness feels potentially at risk himself or herself[34]

By this approach, the person viewed as suffering must be seen as a victim, although the victims themselves may not identify the suffering as serious or even present (eg, a person in a coma evoking compassion from family members), and the compassionate person must be able to identify with the suffering of the other.

Peterson and Seligman[35] include compassion as an important element of the character strength of kindness. Although there is much overlap between compassion and empathy, kindness, sympathy, pity, and altruistic motivation, typical definitions of compassion include these elements as parts of compassion.[36] Strauss and colleagues[36] have reviewed compassion measures. The self-report scales often include items surveying compassion toward familiar and unfamiliar others, toward oneself, and sometimes focus specifically on caregivers (eg, nurses) or the experience of caregiving by patients. Self-compassion, a building block for general compassion, includes a perspective on one's own suffering that encompasses the following:

1. A kind attitude toward oneself
2. Accepting failures as part of life rather than wholly self-induced
3. Maintenance of a balanced, not hyperbolized, narrative of one's suffering[37]

Connection to mental health

Compassion is viewed across cultures and religious traditions as a desirable attribute. Evolutionary biology posits several benefits of this seemingly unproductive trait, including enhancing caregiving toward offspring and kin as well as being an attractive trait in mate selection, as it enhances the ability to cooperate with non-kin.[33–41] Compassion is associated with greater buffering against physiologic reactions to stress,[42] and compassion practice has been shown to produce greater positive emotions[43] and happiness.[44] Higher self-compassion is associated with reduced anxiety, depression, and distress,[45] and with increased positive emotions.[46] In college students, self-compassion correlated with increased happiness, optimism, and other positive traits and was negatively correlated with neuroticism and negative affect.[47]

An hour of weekly compassion training for 6 weeks was shown to increase a variety of positive emotions,[48] which in turn led to increased life satisfaction, positive relationships, and good physical health, as well as fewer depressive symptoms. Even 15 minutes of compassion training demonstrated an increase in positive mood and positive regard for others.[49] Warmth and support by mothers in childhood correlates with both peer-reports and self-reports of compassionate traits across timepoints in adulthood.[50]

Compassionate care is a tenet of major medical organizations.[51,52] Compassion in health care decreases use of emergency department services[53] and lowers spending on diagnostic tests,[54] and may have its greatest cost-saving potential in reducing staff burnout. Psychotherapists and health care workers with higher self-compassion report less burnout.[55,56] A consistently inverse relationship between self-compassion and burnout is reported across clinical mental health staff (social work, psychology, support staff, and psychiatrists).[57]

Growing evidence supports similar findings in adolescents. Adolescents reporting more self-compassion show less stress, and negative affect, and greater life satisfaction.[58] Self-compassion correlated negatively with depression and anxiety, and was associated with more social connectedness.[59]

Highly self-compassionate youth were more satisfied with their lives, less anxious, less depressed, and reported more positive emotions.[60] A meta-analysis showed a large effect size for the relationship between self-compassion and reduced psychological distress (anxiety, depression, stress) in adolescents.[61] School dropouts who were more self-compassionate showed higher self-esteem and lower aggression.[62]

Neuroscience of compassion

The neural basis of compassion overlaps with empathy, kindness, and other humanitarian traits. Hou and colleagues[63] found that compassion overlapped with gray matter volume in empathy circuits, mainly in the anterior insula and anterior cingulate cortex (ACC). Fehse and colleagues[64] found that insula, ACC, and mPFC were activated during compassion toward victims judged to be innocent, rather than responsible for, their own fate. When victims were perceived responsible for their own misfortune, these same brain regions were *de*activated, while activation in dlPFC increased, suggesting a potential compassion network modulated according to the situation. Mascaro and colleagues[65] found that activity in the anterior insula correlated with compassion training. They then focused on empathic accuracy, measured by the ability to identify emotions in others' facial expressions.[66] Empathic accuracy was reliant on increased neural activity in the IFG and dmPFC. This finding implicates compassion practice as a neural workout of sorts, strengthening interpersonal skills often found lacking in those with disorders on the autism or antisocial spectra. Feeling loved by others and the experience of sending love to others may also correspond to self-compassion and general compassion. Both generate activity in closely overlapping areas of ACC and mPFC.[67]

Practices designed to enhance compassion may build neural networks for this trait while bolstering behavioral benefits. Loving kindness meditation involves a "generous" mindset with care toward oneself and loved ones, then extending this to others. Empathy training activates the anterior insula and dorsal ACC, but is associated with negative responses to suffering.[49,57] Compassion training alternately boosted positive emotions to suffering, and this positive affect corresponded with activity in reward-related and compassion-related areas, including the ventral striatum (VS), ventral ACC, and medial OFC. Compared with cognitive reappraisal strategies, compassion practice was more effective overall in increasing positive emotions in response to others' distress, whereas cognitive reappraisal strategies more readily reduced negative emotional responses. Compassion practice correlates with activity increases in reward areas (VS/nucleus accumbens, globus pallidus) and vmPFC, ventral ACC, and mid-insula.[68] Additional fMRI data show differential activation of the inferior parietal cortex and dlPFC in concert with more altruistic giving in the behavioral task by participants trained in compassion. Reappraisal trainees did not show these specific increases in brain activity. Further, connectivity between the dlPFC and the nucleus accumbens predicted more altruistic behavior in compassion trainees.[69] This suggests that compassion training may have benefits for caregivers facing burnout.

SUMMARY

A small portion of neuroscience research on 2 positive traits, optimism and compassion, has been reviewed. Functional neuroimaging studies consistently show activity in the medial prefrontal cortex, anterior insula, OFC, and ACC.[70] Pathways in these regions further interact with reward and executive function centers. Biomarkers may help differentiate those who could most benefit from cultivating certain positive traits and the density of training required. Longitudinal imaging studies may generate knowledge regarding the developmental trajectory of positive trait development and important windows for intervening.

The benefits to emotional and behavioral health derived from targeted application of these traits is becoming increasingly clear. Still, the nuances of how best to promote these traits warrants further study. For example, what are the most effective ways to build positive traits at differing developmental stages? Would universal health promotion efforts to build positive traits be useful and cost-effective, and if so where would be the delivery point? What is the appropriate dose and duration of training? At the secondary and tertiary prevention levels, even less is known about for whom training in positive traits would be appropriate and how it would best be implemented.

The notion of prescribing compassion practice, optimism exercises, and other positive traits and then measuring improvements in well-being in youth and families is compelling. The scientific support for well-being and brain health can now be added to the argument for enhancing compassion in psychiatric work: health promotion, illness prevention, and intervention. That is, building compassion in parents and children holds promise for nurturing positive traits and relationships and creating a foundation for the positive parenting practices that have a great deal of empirical support for fostering healthy families and development. In addition, biomarkers of compassion and its subcomponents may serve to identify those at risk for emotional and behavioral difficulties, resulting in earlier and more targeted referral to appropriate supports, which may include compassion practice. Finally, nurturing compassion in those with identified deficits, such as autism, conduct disorder, and anxiety, may reduce pathology by strengthening neural circuitry that supports positive emotions and social connections needed to overcome these vulnerabilities.

REFERENCES

1. F Crane (1914 January 01, Syracuse Herald, New Year's Resolutions by Dr. Frank Crane, Unnumbered Page (NewsArch Page 16), Column 4, Syracuse, New York. (NewspaperArchive); see Available at: https://quoteinvestigator.com/2012/10/20/happy-minds/#return-note-4604-2).
2. Insel T. Psychiatry as a clinical neuroscience discipline. JAMA 2005;294(17): 2221–4.
3. The Accreditation Council for Graduate Medical Education and The American Board of Psychiatry and Neurology. The Child & Adolescent Psychiatry Milestone Project. 2015. Available at: http://www.acgme.org/Portals/0/PDFs/Milestones/ChildandAdolescentPsychiatryMilestones.pdf. Accessed August 10, 2018.
4. American Academy of Child and Adolescent Psychiatry. Child and adolescent psychiatrists. American Academy of Child and Adolescent Psychiatry Web site. 2015. Available at: https://www.aacap.org/AACAP/Families_and_Youth/Facts_for_Families/FFF-Guide/The-Child-And-Adolescent-Psychiatrist-000.aspx. Accessed August 10, 2018.
5. Seligman MEP, Csikszentmihalyi M. Positive psychology: an introduction. Am Psychol 2000;55:5–14.
6. Hudziak J, Ivanova M. The Vermont family based approach: family based health promotion, illness prevention, and intervention. Child Adolesc Psychiatr Clin N Am 2016;25(2):167–78.
7. Jeste DV, Palmer BW. Positive psychiatry: a clinical handbook. 1st edition. Arlington (VA): American Psychiatric Publishing; 2015.
8. Schlechter A. The positive approach to the diagnostic interview: is talking about what's wrong necessarily right? J Am Acad Child Adolesc Psychiatry 2016; 55(10):S94.
9. Seligman MEP. Authentic happiness: using the new positive psychology to realize your potential for lasting fulfillment. New York: Free Press; 2002.
10. Seligman MEP, Rashid T, Parks AC. Positive psychotherapy. Am Psychol 2006;61: 774–88.
11. Peterson C, Semmel A, von Baeyer C, et al. The attributional style questionnaire. Cognit Ther Res 1982;6(3):287–300.
12. Emmons RA, McCullough ME. Counting blessings versus burdens: an experimental investigation of gratitude and subjective well-being in daily life. J Pers Soc Psychol 2003;84(2):377–89.
13. Dicke A, Hendrick C. The relationship assessment scale. J Soc Pers Relat 1998; 15:137–42.
14. Carver CS, Scheier MF, Miller CJ, et al. Optimism. In: Lopez SJ, Snyder CR, editors. Oxford handbook of positive psychology. 2nd edition. New York: Oxford University Press; 2009. p. 303–11.
15. Kim ES, Hagan KA, Grodstein F, et al. Optimism and cause-specific mortality: a prospective cohort study. Am J Epidemiol 2016;185(1):21–9.

16. Radcliffe NM, Klein WMP. Dispositional, unrealistic, and comparative optimism: differential relations with the knowledge and processing of risk information and beliefs about personal risk. Pers Soc Psychol Bull 2002;28:836–46.
17. Shepperd JA, Maroto JJ, Pbert LA. Dispositional optimism as a predictor of health changes among cardiac patients. J Res Pers 1996;30:517–34.
18. Taylor SE, Kemeny ME, Aspinwall LG, et al. Optimism, coping, psychological distress, and high-risk sexual behavior among men at risk for acquired immuno-deficiency syndrome. J Pers Soc Psychol 1992;63:460–73.
19. Leung BW, Moneta GB, McBride-Chang C. Think positively and feel positively: optimism and life satisfaction in late life. Int J Aging Hum Dev 2005;61(4):335–65.
20. Gallagher MW, Lopez SJ, Pressman SD. Optimism is universal: exploring the presence and benefits of optimism in a representative sample of the world. J Pers 2013;81(5):429–40.
21. Alessandri G, De Pascalis V. Double dissociation between the neural correlates of the general and specific factors of the Life Orientation Test–Revised. Cogn Affect Behav Neurosci 2017;17(5):917.
22. Sharot T, Korn CW, Dolan RJ. How unrealistic optimism is maintained in the face of reality. Nat Neurosci 2011;14(11):1475–9.
23. Sharot T, Guitart-Masip M, Korn CW, et al. How dopamine enhances an optimism bias in humans. Curr Biol 2012;22(16):1477–81.
24. Kuzmanovic B, Jefferson A, Vogeley K. The role of the neural reward circuitry in self-referential optimistic belief updates. Neuroimage 2016;133:151–62.
25. Blair KS, Otero M, Teng C, et al. Dissociable roles of ventromedial prefrontal cortex and rostral anterior cortex in value representation and optimistic bias. Neuroimage 2013;78:103–10.
26. Dolcos S, Hu Y, Iordan AD, et al. Optimism and the brain: trait optimism mediates the protective role of the orbitofrontal cortex gray matter volume against anxiety. Soc Cogn Affect Neurosci 2015;11(2):263–71.
27. Wu J, Dong D, Jackson T, et al. The neural correlates of optimistic and depressive tendencies of self-evaluations and resting-state default mode network. Front Hum Neurosci 2015;9(618):1–11.
28. Blair K, Otero M, Teng C, et al. Reduced optimism and a heightened neural response to everyday worries are specific to generalized anxiety disorder, and not seen in social anxiety. Psychol Med 2017;47(10):1806–15.
29. Garrett N, Sharot T, Faulkner P, et al. Losing the rose tinted glasses: neural substrates of unbiased belief updating in depression. Front Hum Neurosci 2014;8:639.
30. Seligman MEP, Castellon C, Cacciola J, et al. Explanatory style change during cognitive therapy for unipolar depression. J Abnorm Psychol 1988;97(1):13–8.
31. Gillham JE, Reivich KJ, Jaycox LH, et al. Prevention of depressive symptoms in schoolchildren: two-year follow-up. Psychol Sci 1995;6(6):343–51.
32. Reivich K, Gillham JE, Chaplin TM, et al. From helplessness to optimism: the role of resilience in treating and preventing depression in youth. In: Goldstein S, Brooks RB, editors. Handbook of resilience in children. New York: Kluwer Academic/Plenum Publishers; 2005. p. 223–37.
33. Gillham JE, Hamilton J, Freres DR, et al. Preventing depression among early adolescents in the primary care setting: a randomized controlled study of the Penn Resiliency Program. J Abnorm Child Psychol 2006;34(2):203–19.
34. Cassell EJ. Compassion.. In: Lopez SJ, Snyder CR, editors. Oxford handbook of positive psychology. 2nd edition. New York: Oxford University Press; 2009. p. 393–403.

35. Peterson C, Seligman MEP. Character strengths and virtues: a handbook and classification. 1st edition. New York: Oxford University Press; 2004.
36. Strauss C, Taylor BL, Gu J, et al. What is compassion and how can we measure it? A review of definitions and measures. Clin Psychol Rev 2016;47:15–27.
37. Neff KD. The development and validation of a scale to measure self-compassion. Self Ident 2003;2:223–50.
38. Gilbert P. Compassion and cruelty: a biopsychosocial approach. In: Gilbert P, editor. Compassion: conceptualisations, research and use in psychotherapy. London: Routledge; 2005. p. 9–74.
39. Goetz JL, Keltner D, Simon-Thomas E. Compassion: an evolutionary analysis and empirical review. Psychol Bull 2010;136(3):351–74.
40. de Waal F. The age of empathy. New York: Harmony; 2009.
41. Keltner D. Born to be good: the science of a meaningful life. New York: Norton; 2009.
42. Cosley BJ, McCoy SK, Saslow LR, et al. Is compassion for others stress buffering? Consequences of compassion and social support for physiological reactivity to stress. J Exp Soc Psychol 2010;46:816–23.
43. Klimecki OM, Leiberg S, Lamm C, et al. Functional neural plasticity and associated changes in positive affect after compassion training. Cereb Cortex 2013; 23(7):1552–61.
44. Mongrain M, Chin JM, Shapira L. Practicing compassion increases happiness and self-esteem. J Happiness Stud 2011;12:963–81.
45. MacBeth A, Gumley A. Exploring compassion: a meta-analysis of the association between self-compassion and psychopathology. Clin Psychol Rev 2012;32(6): 545–52.
46. López A, Sanderman R, Ranchor AV, et al. Compassion for others and self-compassion: levels, correlates, and relationship with psychological well-being. Mindfulness (N Y) 2018;9(1):325.
47. Neff KD, Rude SS, Kirkpatrick KL. An examination of self-compassion in relation to positive psychological functioning and personality traits. J Res Pers 2007;41: 908–16.
48. Fredrickson BL, Cohn MA, Coffey KA, et al. Open hearts build lives: positive emotions, induced through loving-kindness meditation, build consequential personal resources. J Pers Soc Psychol 2008;95(5):1045–62.
49. Hutcherson CA, Seppala EM, Gross JJ. Loving-kindness meditation increases social connectedness. Emotion 2008;8(5):720–4.
50. Eisenberg N, VanSchyndel SK, Hofer C. The association of maternal socialization in childhood and adolescence with adult offsprings' sympathy/caring. Dev Psychol 2015;51(1):7–16.
51. American Medical Association. AMA code of medical ethics. 2001. Available at: https://www.ama-assn.org/sites/default/files/media-browser/principles-of-medical-ethics.pdf Copyright 2016. Accessed August 13, 2018.
52. National Health Service, Department of Health. The handbook to the NHS constitution. 2015. Available at: https://assets.publishing.service.gov.uk/government/uploads/system/uploads/attachment_data/file/474450/NHS_Constitution_Handbook_v2.pdf. Accessed August 13, 2018.
53. Redelmeier DA, Molin JP, Tibshirani RJ. A randomised trial of compassionate care for the homeless in an emergency department. Lancet 1995;345(8958): 1131–4.
54. Epstein RM, Franks P, Shields CG, et al. Patient-centered communication and diagnostic testing. Ann Fam Med 2005;3(5):415–21.

55. Beaumont E, Durkin M, Hollins Martin CJ, et al. Measuring relationships between self-compassion, compassion fatigue, burnout and well-being in student counsellors and student cognitive behavioural psychotherapists: a quantitative survey. Couns Psychother Res 2016;16(1). https://doi.org/10.1002/capr.12054.
56. Scarlet J, Altmeyer N, Knier S, et al. The effects of Compassion Cultivation Training (CCT) on health-care workers. Clin Psychol 2017;21(2). https://doi.org/10.1111/cp.12130.
57. Atkinson DM, Rodman JL, Thuras PD, et al. Examining burnout, depression, and self-compassion in Veterans Affairs mental health staff. J Altern Complement Med 2017;23(7):551–7.
58. Bluth K, Blanton PW. The influence of self-compassion on emotional well-being among early and older adolescent males and females. J Posit Psychol 2015; 10(3):219–30.
59. Neff KD, McGehee P. Self-compassion and psychological resilience among adolescents and young adults. Self Ident 2010;9(3):225–40.
60. Bluth K, Roberson PN, Gaylord SA, et al. Does self-compassion protect adolescents from stress? J Child Fam Stud 2016;25(4):1098–109.
61. Marsh IC, Chan SWY, MacBeth A. Self-compassion and psychological distress in adolescents—a meta-analysis. Mindfulness (N Y) 2018;9:1011.
62. Barry CT, Loflin DC, Doucette H. Adolescent self-compassion: associations with narcissism, self-esteem, aggression, and internalizing symptoms in at-risk males. Pers Indiv Differ 2015;77:118–23.
63. Hou X, Allen TA, Wei D, et al. Trait compassion is associated with the neural substrate of empathy. Cogn Affect Behav Neurosci 2017;17:1018.
64. Fehse K, Silveira S, Elvers K, et al. Compassion, guilt and innocence: an fMRI study of responses to victims who are responsible for their fate. Soc Neurosci 2015;10(3):243–52.
65. Mascaro JS, Rilling JK, Negi LT, et al. Pre-existing brain function predicts subsequent practice of mindfulness and compassion meditation. Neuroimage 2013;69:35–42.
66. Mascaro JS, Rilling JK, Negi LT, et al. Compassion meditation enhances empathic accuracy and related neural activity. Soc Cogn Affect Neurosci 2013; 8(1):48–55.
67. Hutcherson CA, Seppala EM, Gross JJ. The neural correlates of social connection. Cogn Affect Behav Neurosci 2015;15(1):1–14.
68. Engen HG, Singer T. Compassion-based emotion regulation up-regulates experienced positive affect and associated neural networks. Social Cogn Affective Neurosci 2015;10(9):1291–301.
69. Weng HY, Fox AS, Shackman AJ, et al. Compassion training alters altruism and neural responses to suffering. Psychol Sci 2013;24(7):1171–80.
70. Moore RC, Eyler LT, Mills PJ, et al. Biology of positive psychiatry. In: Jeste DV, Palmer BW, editors. Positive psychiatry: a clinical handbook. Arlington (VA): American Psychiatric Publishing; 2015. p. 261–83.

Happiness When the Body Hurts

Achieving Well-Being in Chronic Health Conditions

Megan McCormick, PhD[a],*, Grace Cushman, MS[b]

KEYWORDS

- Well-being • Chronic • Illness • PERMA • IBD • Happiness • GI

KEY POINTS

- Children can find a sense of well-being even in the midst of chronic illness.
- Adult caregivers can help to guide youth in reframing *happiness*.
- PERMA provides a model through which youth can thrive and flourish when experiencing ongoing challenges.

OVERCOMING THE ODDS

One of humanity's most prevailing and widely embraced narratives is overcoming adversity. We all welcome the stories of underdogs conquering the unthinkable with focus, determination, and "heart" (whatever that is). Scientifically, the evidence does not suggest otherwise. The architecture of our brains and bodies are constructed to endure time-limited stress and return to a healthy baseline.[1] People run ultramarathons, endure tense conversation with bosses, and survive brutal traffic commutes. However, the chronic physical conditions, that do not offer a guaranteed end, and with no course promising relief, yield a much less satisfying story. It is difficult to hear the inspiring soundtrack in the background, and it is not an option to merely grit your teeth, shut out the world, and dissociate to run to a finish line.

Chronic illnesses, such as type 1 diabetes, chronic kidney disease, or inflammatory bowel disease (IBD), threaten our traditional notions of *happiness* (eg, comfort, health, normalcy). For youth, in particular, chronic illness can further complicate universally arduous developmental milestones: solidifying an individual identity,

Disclosure Statement: The authors have nothing to disclose.
[a] Georgetown University, 2115 Wisconsin Avenue Northwest, Suite 200, Washington, DC 20007, USA; [b] University of Georgia, 125 Baldwin Street, Athens, GA 30602, USA
* Corresponding author.
E-mail address: megan.l.mccormick@gunet.georgetown.edu

Child Adolesc Psychiatric Clin N Am 28 (2019) 147–156
https://doi.org/10.1016/j.chc.2018.11.008
1056-4993/19/© 2018 Elsevier Inc. All rights reserved.

connecting with likeminded peers, pursuing romantic interests, and transitioning toward independent living.[2] In addition, young brains lack the fully developed executive functions that assist with such challenges. To think flexibly, take perspective, organize thoughts, and accurately weigh the gravity of experiences are still developing into early adulthood.

So how can a child live a happy life while facing a persistent and recurrent hardship like chronic disease? A different notion of "happiness" is required: "The goal of positive psychology in *well-being theory* (is not to increase the amount of happiness)...but to increase the amount of *flourishing* in your own life and on the planet."[3] Well-being is holistic, cumulative, and enduring, and it can exist even when we are not comfortable, healthy, or seemingly "normal." In this article, Seligman's PERMA theory of well-being[3] is applied to childhood chronic illness, providing direction for a different narrative that promotes emotional, cognitive, and social prosperity against the odds. This article uses IBD as the example for integrating well-being practices, but these principles also apply to other chronic health conditions.

Inflammatory Bowel Disease

Adolescence is a time filled with questions about identity and meaning and sometimes feeling lost. For those youth with a chronic medical condition like IBD, a diminished sense of control over their lives and future, as well as feeling vulnerable and different from others their age, is particularly salient.[4] The symptoms of IBD may contribute to a lack of well-being and feeling as though life is beyond their control. Many youth with IBD are plagued with uncomfortable and painful inflammation of the gastrointestinal tract, which can cause abdominal pain, fever, fatigue, diarrhea, hematochezia, weight loss, and growth delays .[5,6] This inflammation is often episodic and can be unpredictable as patients undergo periods of active disease and remission. The exact cause of IBD remains unclear, but appears tied to interactions of environmental, genetic, and immune factors; yet the exact cause remains unclear.[5] Therefore, it is difficult to determine when and where these youth may experience flare-ups. Having unexpected bowel movements, flatulence, intense physical discomfort, and limitations on diet are also common experiences in IBD. Growth can also be stunted, causing patients to appear shorter and smaller than their peers.

In addition to the physical symptoms themselves, the interventions for IBD can be intrusive and disruptive to daily living. Shortly after diagnosis, many youth are prescribed corticosteroids (eg, prednisone), aminosalicylates (eg, 5-aminosalicylate), immunomodulators (eg, 6-MP), or biologics (eg, infliximab).[7,8] Although studies have shown them to be effective in decreasing the severity of symptoms, negative and embarrassing side effects can occur (eg, facial swelling).[8] Also, many patients have to undergo infusion-based treatments such as infliximab, which are time intensive and can only be delivered in medical offices.[9,10]

The negative experience of having a chronic illness goes beyond just the physical symptoms. Severe cases of ulcerative colitis and Crohn disease, 2 diseases within the IBD category, are sometimes treated with surgeries and procedures. Removal of part or all of the colon, rectum, or anus can occur and are among the most invasive procedures.[11] Some youth may also need ileostomy or colostomy bags to catch waste if their bodies are unable to eliminate it after removal of parts of the gastrointestinal system.[11]

In addition to medication and medical interventions, basic lifestyle changes are also required to manage symptoms. In order to prevent flare-ups of symptoms, youth are recommended to adhere to an atypical adolescent routine of a strict sleep schedule, avoiding alcohol, eating healthy, and reducing stress as much as possible.[12] Although many of these lifestyle characteristics are recommended for all adolescents, youth with IBD must adherent more than their peers to reduce the likelihood of flare-ups.

PERMA as Applied to Inflammatory Bowel Disease

For each of the components of PERMA, relevant IBD-specific considerations are examined, as well as concrete strategies for activating each ingredient of Seligman's model to achieve well-being in youth with IBD. Sample questions and action steps for including PERMA into interviews of patients with chronic illnesses are summarized in **Table 1**.

P: Positive emotion

It is easy to imagine the inevitable negative emotions felt by youth diagnosed with IBD *and* their caregivers. The initial experience of receiving a diagnosis of a chronic illness can be psychologically similar to mourning the loss of a loved one.[13] For many, the relief of uncovering the cause of their child's sickness is quickly overshadowed by feelings of shock, denial, and grief, as both youth and their parents mourn the loss of a "normal life." In addition, daily life with IBD breeds additional negative emotion. Unpredictable flare-ups cause anxiety and fear; symptoms and medication side effects cause embarrassment, and missed activities cause disappointment. Feelings of shame, guilt, and envy are also palpable, as the normative mindset of youth leaves them asking the questions, *"Why me? What did I do to deserve this?,"* and the evolutionary need to protect our young causes parents to fret, *"Could I have prevented this? Genetically did I bring this on my child? Did I do something during the pregnancy to cause this? My friends complaining about travel sports schedules for their children perturb me—they don't know how lucky they are to have healthy children."*

The first step is to alter the usual chase for *happiness* and embrace a *well-being* mindset. Peace, fulfillment, serenity, joy, inspiration, gratitude, and awe are accessible experiences for youth living with chronic illness, even amid temporary pain, sadness, or uncertainty.[14] Second, negative emotions do not always necessitate feelings of *distress*. Feelings alone are temporary providing no direct harm. Adolescents may feel lonely one night when a friend forgets them, but feel excited the next morning when the same friend calls. Attaching judgment to negative emotions: *"I've inherited my mother's depression," "I'll be alone forever," "I shouldn't be feeling this upset,"* fosters distress, perpetuating and exacerbating the experience of negative emotions.[15]

Although humans seek to protect others from feeling badly,[16] attempting to "fix" a young person's negative feelings about chronic illness can be invalidating and unhelpful. Encouraging *"Just think happy thoughts!"* or sending smiling emojis can send the message, *"You shouldn't be feeling this way."* Guiding youth to positive emotion requires tact, patience, and a genuine demonstration of the mentality you hope to cultivate. Instead of rushing to make the negative emotion go away, the brain can be taught that negative emotion and positive well-being can co-exist. Give permission to have negative feelings (*"It makes sense that you would feel worried"*), adopt a personal mantra (*"Feelings come and go, like waves, and he'll/I'll be okay"*), and offer choices to restore control (*"We can talk [write/draw] about it, or we can let the feeling pass through you"*). Negative emotions indeed alert us that we may want to reconsider our current course, that what we are doing does not *feel* right.

Cognitive behavioral therapy (CBT) and acceptance and commitment therapy (ACT) provide a structured approach to reducing distress through the use of strategies like mindfulness and cognitive diffusion[17]; see *Get Out of Your Life and Into Your Mind* for self-guided learning.[18] Rather than focusing on eliminating mental health symptoms or triggers, ACT encourages a person to make change in their life without first changing

Table 1
PERMA and chronic illness

	Positive Emotions (P)	Engagement (E)	Relationships (R)	Meaning (M)	Accomplishment (A)
Description	Cultivating peace, fulfillment, serenity, joy, inspiration, and gratitude	Staying active, finding new ways to engage with others or the community	Support from and connection with others	Finding purpose, belongingness, and meaning with a medical illness	Mastery or competence in subjective experiences
Eliciting questions for youth living with chronic illness	• How long do your feelings usually last before you feel something else? • Does your condition cause you to feel certain emotions? • Can you feel (fulfillment) even if you're feeling (frustrate)? • How can we "turn down the volume" on that feeling: it will still be there, but it doesn't bother you as much?	• Is it important to you to stay involved and active? • Are there ways you could still sometimes do the activities you like? • Can you participate in other ways? • Is there something new you've been wanting to try that you could still do now? • Are you able to "lose yourself" during certain activities?	• Do you think it is helpful to have support from others? • How has this condition affected your friendships? • How do friends treat you now? • How can you still spend time with friends even when you're feeling sick? • Even though it would be hard, could it be helpful to share your diagnosis with a few friends?	• What does this illness mean to you? How does it define you, and how does it not? • How is life different before and after you were diagnosed? • What unique perspective do you have now that others may not have? • Could this illness make something in your life better? • How much time does your condition take up in your life?	• What activities give you a sense of accomplishment? How could you do a little bit every day? • Little things like (taking your medication) are accomplishments; could we track those each day? • Do you have other goals (do a new activity, more time with friends, and so forth) that you want to pursue?
Action items for adults working with youth living with chronic illness	• Try to "stay with" negative feelings before examining options for changes • Empower youth to talk/write about feelings, or to "let negative feelings pass like a wave" • Encourage mental health support (CBT, ACT)	• Recognize warning signs of disengagement • Validate that engagement may have to change, but encourage as much engagement as possible within limitations of illness	• Collaboratively brainstorm ways to stay connected • Help generate and practice a brief speech (3 sentences) to tell others about diagnosis	• Encourage discussion about diagnosis and how it fits into their "life story" • Seek out others who have similar diagnosis (or understand through relatives and others) through support groups, social media, or camps	• Foster a sense of control, mastery, or pride • Encourage setting new/feasible goals • Visually track accomplishments (eg, white boards, lists, charts)

negative feelings or circumstances. By practicing acceptance, identifying realistic targets for internal change, and using individual values (eg, fulfillment) to guide and gauge progress, patients can adopt a more expedient, stable pathway toward relief, and more useful for chronic illness populations. Accepting and embracing the inevitability of negative emotions decreases the power of these emotions and prepares for positive well-being.

E: Engagement

Many youth may have been functioning normally before diagnosis of IBD. They may have attended school regularly, participated in activities such as sports teams, or attended religious/spiritual gatherings. Engaging with their immediate environment, community, and those around them may have been normal in their development. However, painful or embarrassing physical symptoms often restrict social activities and create isolation, even before IBD is identified.[19] This diagnostic process can be slow, and disengagement may also look different for every child or resemble "normal teenage behavior," making it easy to miss the warning signs.

When IBD is officially diagnosed, immediate questions like *"Can I still play basketball?* and *"What about my debate team trip?"* are common. Although sometimes frustrating for parents, *"Please focus on your health right now!,"* these indicate the strong need for youth to feel engaged in their surroundings. Furthermore, youth may see a diagnosis as confirming that they are becoming ever more different from peers. This potential lack of belongingness may perpetuate further disengagement and resignation to protect themselves from additional anxiety.

> Case Example: Chloe is a high school sophomore and member of the track team. At the beginning of the fall semester, she began to experience unpredictable, painful IBD symptoms, but still competed in the first 2 track meets, but performed less well. During one practice, she had to sprint to the bathroom as she felt the onset of diarrhea. Missed practices became more common, and Chloe was told she could not compete in the next track meet due to missing practice. Although saddened at losing her role on the team, she felt relieved from the anxiety of not knowing what might suddenly occur in front of others. Chloe decided to withdraw from the team.

Although quitting the track team may have seemed necessary to Chloe, youth can remain engaged with peers and community. They may not be able to participate in all activities, but they may participate in many familiar activities despite their illness. In addition, new opportunities for engagement (eg, afterschool club, photography, school newspaper) can be introduced that may engage Chloe with peers like the lost activity. Parents can also help children think of ways to continue engaging their same activities but in a different form (track team manager or photographer). Chloe may not be able to compete if she is experiencing a flare-up in symptoms, but she may be able to serve other functions, so that she can see remain a valued part of the team.

A shift in thinking from *"I can't do that anymore"* to *"My course is to do this other activity"* may help sustain engagement. Motivational interviewing techniques are effective to reduce ambivalence and create more lasting changes in thinking and behaviors.[20] Motivation for change is elicited from within the individual, not imposed from the outside, and is particularly useful in adolescents.[21] Parents can model and reinforce the child for using *can* language instead of *can't* language to increase positive thinking around engagement, and to enhance a positive sense of identity and belongingness. Vital to this engagement process is finding alternatives to replace prior activities, and optimally, where the youth becomes so engaged so as to "lose track of time." High engagement fosters the quest for finding activities whereby complete immersion occurs, an approach valuable for everyone as they grow and change.

R: Relationships

Support from friends, family, and peers is invaluable during times of stress. Emotional social support can help people recover from loss or grief and accelerate their return to healthier functioning.[22] Important relationships also provide clarity as to an individual's purpose or meaning in life, because relationships are integral in one's individualism.[23] Within the context of a pediatric chronic illness, social support has been associated with beneficial disease adaptation for chronically ill youth.[24] For those with IBD, however, it may be difficult to lean on their friends in their time of need. Because symptoms of pediatric IBD can be painful or embarrassing, pediatric patients may be uncomfortable disclosing their diagnosis or symptoms for fear of losing friends. They may also worry about rumors, bullying, or pity from a "sick kid" identity at school. These children and adolescents may avoid friends and increasingly isolate themselves. This avoidance pattern perpetuates the cycle of disengagement, detracts from this important identity stage in their development, and estranges them from one of the richest sources of positive well-being during hardship.

A diagnosis of a chronic illness like IBD can make a young individual question the world's ability to accept them, leading to feelings of shame and social avoidance. Despite their child's urges to retreat from friends, parents should recognize this avoidance as based in fear and reinforce that the illness has not changed the child's ability to engage in relationships or altered their likable characteristics. Caregivers can help children sustain current relationships by helping the child think of activities they can still do with friends during flare-ups (eg, watching movies at home). They can also encourage new friendships with youth who may be experiencing similar difficulties. For those interested in meeting others who are diagnosed with IBD, support groups, peer mentors, and summer camps can be identified with the help of their medical team. Many disease-specific foundations (eg, Crohn's and Colitis Foundation) also offer ways for youth to connect with others experiencing similar issues.

Caregivers can help their child discuss disclosing their condition to trusted friends (eg, "They can support you; they can do activities that you are comfortable with and able to do") as well as consequences of withholding (eg, "They won't be able to support you and may misunderstand why you are not around or think you don't like them anymore"). Youth benefit from adult input while navigating such daunting and unfamiliar situations. The child can compose and practice a short (30-second) description about their illness to use when ready to disclose to others. Having a practiced description of their illness lessens their immediate fears and becomes a tool for life. It is important to allow each individual to control the level of detail disclosed; for some, that may be as simple as, "I have a medical condition, so sometimes my body feels sick and I have to miss school." Every person goes at their own pace, and this is particularly relevant when a youth is derailed from future aspirations by learning about a chronic condition that may alter their plans.

M: Meaning

Seligman once wrote, "Positive emotion alienated from the exercise of character leads to emptiness, inauthenticity, depression, and, as we age, the gnawing realization that we are fidgeting until we die."[25] Seligman conveys a critical truth about happiness and about his own model of well-being: that there are no shortcuts to true happiness, and even positive emotion is worth little when there is no *meaning*. Everyone has experienced the instantaneous cognitive reaction that often follows an unexpected realization: "*What does this mean?*" The brain attempts to find meaning in every moment, and naturally associates, categorizes, and attempts to make sense of every experience. By utilizing these cognitive skills, the brain efficiently organizes and integrates information to help one make good decisions and move away from danger and toward well-being. However, when the information does not fit somewhere or make sense (fit a *schema*[26]), one can feel frozen, confused, paralyzed, and searching for how this information or experience fits into one's life.

A diagnosis of chronic illness inevitably elicits the existential question, "*What does this mean?*" Given the rare incidence of childhood chronic illness, most people do not have a context or paradigm for understanding it, and the discordance can cause uncertainty, panic, or depression. Many youth with chronic illness and their families attempt to keep this part of their lives compartmentalized. Worried that IBD will "define" them, many families limit conversation about the disease to only what is necessary: appointments, symptom checks, "Did you take your medicine?" Unfortunately, this approach can work against well-being, because it does not allow the child or family to create a story that the brain can understand and integrate into its larger sense of meaning.

What a disease like IBD *means* to an individual often takes many forms over time. However, parents and caregivers can implement a useful paradigm for a child in this process. First, simply stating the questions everyone knows (but may not want to admit) are in the minds of young patients models courage: "*What does this mean for my future? How does this fit into my life? Will I still accomplish my goals? Who am I, now that I have this? How will this really alter the minutes of my life?*" For adolescents, these questions are developmentally germane, but many of them need adults to sanction and give words to their worries. Caregivers must also resist the urge to quickly reassure the child that "nothing will change." Instead, encouraging youth to "write their story" (narrative) about chronic illnesses like IBD may help them see their progress. Stories are a critical vehicle through which all humans learn, comprehend, and share. When a child takes time to write out their experiences of being diagnosed and living with IBD, they are better able to organize their thoughts and feelings into a story that is meaningful. Furthermore, this narrative becomes a way that they can talk and think about the disease more easily, and the resulting increase in *exposure* to this otherwise difficult topic can reduce worry and distress, as it does for anxiety and trauma.[27]

It is also helpful to explore external ways that youth can begin to think of their disease as something that could, at times, help them or others (altruism). Whether participating in research or raising money for efforts to cure a disease, educating others to increase awareness and reduce stigma, guiding one's career path, or merely gaining perspective about "not sweating the small stuff," finding meaning in each person's unique struggle can illuminate meaning and enhance well-being.

Finally, meaning is perhaps best measured by how one spends their minutes. Although a debilitating chronic illness, such as IBD, may steal time away from the youth's interests, it also requires the person to consider what is truly valued, which activities are more important, and to continue to build those into the minutes of one's daily life (in Chloe's case, making music to share with others, or a sport such as swimming), to revise meaning in one's life.

A: Accomplishment
The words "*accomplishment*" and "*achievement*" sometimes imply needs for objective success measured by the community (eg, good grades, sports records, or

prestigious college acceptances). Seligman's A, however, captures the broader phenomena of *mastery* or *competence*, which any person can attain. When a toddler stacks a block, a child receives a proud smile from his parent, or a grandmother learns a new phrase in different language, they have experienced mastery. When one feels a sense of accomplishment, a critical message is sent to the brain that is critical for well-being: *"Our actions produce results, and we have the ability to succeed."* Even within small tasks, each time the brain receives this message, our *locus of control* is strengthened and internalized.[28] We recognize we are capable and worthy of making important changes for ourselves and others.

Youth diagnosed with IBD often experience limitations on activities, decreased engagement, and uncertainty about their futures, which can thwart opportunities for mastery. Receiving a diagnosis of chronic illness alone can make a child feel victimized; one is unexpectedly hit with a life-altering message, which inevitably produces feelings of powerlessness and lack of control.[29] Because of this, caregivers must also be aware of this important aspect of well-being and continually help their child or patient find ways to redeem their sense of control, predictability, and mastery.

Setting and attaining goals is a critical part of this process. Accomplishing small goals as a part of momentary, daily life (eg, getting to work on time, fueling our bodies with food and water, sorting the mail). Although rarely seen as accomplishments (given their commonplace occurrence), reframing one's perspective allows these everyday tasks to be viewed as (1) critical to our well-being, and (2) goals to be obtained. In addition, youth can set novel goals and find new opportunities to experience mastery in the context of illness (eg, working a puzzle, researching a concept, cooking dinner). Parents can also increase exposure to activities whereby a child already feels mastery. For example, if the child is a good speller, challenging new words at dinner provides regular reminders of this mastery.

For any of these endeavors, goals that are small and obtainable increase opportunities for mastery to be felt often enough to counterbalance the daily struggles of chronic illness. Goals that can be visibly tracked: using lists, white boards, and so forth, help reinforce these accomplishments. When a young person *sees* achievement of even small goals each day and knows these goals are contributing to a larger sense of well-being, the feeling that *"things happen to me"* pivots to *"I make things happen,"* enhancing the internal locus of control and sense of mastery critical to well-being.

SUMMARY

The position that *"Pain is inevitable, suffering is optional"* may challenge implementation. Beyond the feel-good, legendary tales of triumph over tribulation, notable models, Victor Frankl, Frederick Douglass, or Thich Quang Duc ("The Burning Monk"), prove that greatness can be achieved *amid* hardship when one is willing to modify one's thinking. For affected youth, their families, and even medical practitioners, imagining a happy life amid chronic illness, such as IBD, may not seem viable. Seligman's PERMA model provides an alternative for writing a new narrative. All caregivers, at home, at school, and within a medical team, can act as models and advocates for implementation of these PERMA concepts. Although the approach may differ based on the specific child's needs, in general, promoting flexible and adaptive thinking, communication, and understanding about one's disease helps to redefine how happiness is viewed. Young people facing chronic adversity can feel empowered to adopt a *well-being mindset* that engages, integrates, endures, and thrives in any environment.

REFERENCES

1. Segerstrom SC, Miller GE. Psychological stress and the human immune system: a meta-analytic study of 30 years of inquiry. Psychol Bull 2004;130(4):601–30.
2. Yeo M, Sawyer S. ABC of adolescence: chronic illness and disability. BMJ 2005; 330(7493):721–3.
3. Seligman MEP. Flourish. New York: Simon & Schuster; 2011.
4. Nicholas DB, Otley A, Smith C, et al. Challenges and strategies of children and adolescents with inflammatory bowel disease: a qualitative examination. Health Qual Life Outcomes 2007;5:28–35.
5. Diefenbach KA, Breuer CK. Pediatric inflammatory bowel disease. World J Gastroenterol 2006;12:3204–12.
6. Mackner LM, Sisson DP, Crandall WV. Review: psychosocial issues in pediatric inflammatory bowel disease. J Pediatr Psychol 2004;29:243–57.
7. Borrelli O, Cordischi L, Cirulli M, et al. Polymeric diet alone versus corticosteroids in the treatment of active pediatric crohn's disease: a randomized controlled open-label trial. Clin Gastroenterol Hepatol 2006;4(6):744–53.
8. Sauer CG, Kugathasan S. Pediatric inflammatory bowel disease: highlighting pediatric differences in IBD. Gastroenterol Clin North Am 2009;38(4):611–28.
9. Baldassano R, Braegger CP, Escher JC, et al. Infliximab (REMICADE) therapy in the treatment of pediatric Crohn's disease. Am J Gastroenterol 2003;98(4):833–8.
10. Sandborn WJ, Hanauer SB. Infliximab in the treatment of Crohn's Disease: a user's guide for clinicians. Am J Gastroenterol 2002;97(12):2963–72.
11. Shin CE. Pediatric IBD surgery. In: Bayless TM, Hanaeur SB, editors. Advanced therapy in inflammatory bowel disease. 3rd edition. Shelton (CT): PMPH USA; 2011. p. 807–14.
12. Neuman MG, Nanau RM. Inflammatory bowel disease: role of diet, microbiota, life style. Transl Res 2012;160(1):29–44.
13. Boss P, Couden BA. Ambiguous loss from chronic physical illness: clinical interventions with individuals, couples, and families. J Clin Psychol 2002;58(11): 1351–60.
14. Gable SL, Haidt J. What (and why) is positive psychology? Rev Gen Psychol 2005;9(2):103–10.
15. Kellogg SH, Young JE. Cognitive therapy. In: Lebow JL, editor. Twenty- first century psychotherapies: contemporary approaches to theory and practice. Hoboken (NJ): John Wiley & Sons Inc; 2008. p. 43–79.
16. Al-Shawaf L, Conroy-Beam D, Asao K, et al. Human emotions: an evolutionary psychology perspective. Emot Rev 2015;8(2):173–86.
17. Wetherell JL, Afari N, Rutledge T, et al. A randomized, controlled trial of acceptance and commitment therapy and cognitive-behavioral therapy for chronic pain. Pain 2011;152(9):2098–107.
18. Hayes SC. Get out of your mind and into your life: the new acceptance and commitment therapy. Oakland (CA): New Harbinger Publications; 2005.
19. Meijer SA, Sinnema G, Bijstra JO, et al. Social functioning in children with a chronic illness. J Child Psychol Psychiatry 2000;41(3):309–17.
20. Miller WR, Rollnick S. Motivational interviewing: preparing people to change addictive behavior. New York: Guilford Press; 1991. ISBN 978-0-89862-566-0.
21. Naar-King S, Suarez M. Motivational interviewing with adolescents and young adults. New York: Guilford Press; 2014. ISBN 978-1609180621.
22. Linley PA, Joseph S. Positive change following trauma and adversity: a review. J Trauma Stress 2004;17(1):11–21.

23. Ladd GW. Peer relationships and social competence during early and middle childhood. Annu Rev Psychol 1999;50:333–59.

24. La Greca AM, Bearman KJ, Moore H. Peer relations of youth with pediatric conditions and health risks: promoting social support and healthy lifestyles. J Dev Behav Pediatr 2002;23(4):271–80.

25. Seligman MEP. Authentic happiness: using the new positive psychology to realize your potential for lasting fulfillment. New York: Free Press; 2002.

26. Piaget J. Origins of intelligence in the child. London: Routledge & Kegan Paul; 1936.

27. Foa E, Kozak M. Emotional processing of fear: exposure to corrective information. Psychol Bull 1986;99:20–35.

28. Bandura A. Self-efficacy: the exercise of control. New York: W. H. Freeman; 1997.

29. Meijer SA, Sinnema G, Bijstra JO, et al. Coping styles and locus of control as predictors for psychological adjustment of adolescents with a chronic illness. Soc Sci Med 2002;54(9):1453–61.

Integration into Clinical Psychiatry

The Positive Assessment
A Model for Integrating Well-Being and Strengths-Based Approaches into the Child and Adolescent Psychiatry Clinical Evaluation

Alan Daniel Schlechter, MD[a],*,
Kyle H. O'Brien, PhD, DHSc, MSW, MSOT, LCSW, OTR/L[b],
Colin Stewart, MD[c]

KEYWORDS

- Positive emotions • Positive psychology • Psychiatry interview • Well-being
- Diagnostic interview • Assessment • Rapport • Common factors theory

KEY POINTS

- The traditional psychiatric interview that has been used for the past 80 years is based on the medical model and has no evidence base to support that its structure encourages rapport, diagnosis, or treatment.
- Negative and positive emotions have different purposes. Eliciting positive emotions encourages trust, compromise, and many other qualities that are ideal for developing rapport with the patient.
- The current psychiatric interview proceeds directly to assessing the negative emotions of a patient, but a positive assessment would begin with a study of the patient's strengths and then proceed to understanding the patient's challenges.
- By assessing the strengths of a patient, the clinician may elicit positive emotions from the caregiver and patient, which facilitates rapport, diagnosis, and treatment.
- The diagnostic interview should be modified and vigorously tested to ensure that it is ideally suited for helping develop rapport, eliciting symptoms, and aiding in diagnosis and treatment.

Disclosure Statement: None of the authors have any direct financial interests in subject matter or materials discussed in the article or with a company making a competing product.
[a] Department of Child and Adolescent Psychiatry, Outpatient Child and Adolescent Psychiatry, NYU Langone Health, Bellevue Hospital, Hassenfeld Children's Hospital at NYU Langone, Child Study Center, 462 First Avenue, Room A244, New York, NY 10016, USA; [b] Department of Social Work, Southern Connecticut State University, 101 Farnham Avenue, Office 114, New Haven, CT 06515, USA; [c] Child and Adolescent Psychiatry, Georgetown University Medical Center, School of Medicine, 2115 Wisconsin Avenue Northwest, Suite 200, Washington, DC 20007, USA
* Corresponding author.
E-mail address: alan.schlechter@nyumc.org

Child Adolesc Psychiatric Clin N Am 28 (2019) 157–169
https://doi.org/10.1016/j.chc.2018.11.009
childpsych.theclinics.com

In traditional general medical practice, the diagnostic interview is focused on symptom collection, diagnosis, and treatment. The general medical interview has many tools at its disposal: the physical examination, laboratory tests, radiologic studies, and numerous other means of ascertaining clinical signs and symptoms. Medical and surgical doctors are encouraged to develop rapport with the patient, but many patients who have commented on the terrible bedside manner of a doctor still seek out that physician because of reputation and perceived expertise.[1] Psychiatry has used the same general medical model for its diagnostic interview. Chief complaint, history of present illness, past history, developmental history, family history, and a mental status examination have been collected by residents in training in compliance with the American Board of Psychiatry and Neurology for more than 80 years (the Child and Adolescent examination was created in 1959). Although the psychiatric interview is based on the medical model, psychiatrists typically rely less on laboratory and imaging findings to guide diagnosis and treatment. History and examination therefore carry special importance in psychiatry, and rapport is a critical factor in optimizing information obtained from the patient. Rapport is among the most essential tools for the psychiatrist to discern significant, sometimes patient-minimized, symptoms, to develop a diagnosis and a treatment plan.[2]

There are many modalities of psychotherapy, but common factors theory proposes that regardless of the type of psychotherapy, specific shared qualities determine a successful treatment. Lambert[2] found four components essential to a successful outcome:

- The patient's desire to change (40%)
- The quality of the rapport (30%)
- The positive expectancy of the patient (15%)
- The therapist's skill (15%)

During the diagnostic interview, the therapist brings clinical skills, but more importantly has the opportunity to influence that patient's desire to change, the quality of the rapport, and the positive expectancy. The current structure of the psychiatric interview, which is solution-focused, may be the simplest way to quickly collect the symptoms of the patient, yet may not be optimally organized to support these "common factors" that lead to successful treatment outcomes.

If developing rapport is essential to the successful psychiatric diagnostic interview, then a different interview format may be needed to facilitate this process. We propose that a "positive assessment" that elicits information about the patient's well-being and strengths at the outset of the interview may provide such a format. Although the traditional interview is designed to rapidly elicit negative symptoms at the outset to focus the interview, this strategy may inhibit the development of rapport, thereby interfering with optimal diagnosis and treatment. Discussing the patient's strengths and well-being is more likely to encourage trust, compromise, hope, and a desire to change. The last 30 years have seen the development of scientific studies and evidenced-based practices that draw on findings from positive psychology. We advance an evidenced-based rationale for the positive assessment in the psychiatric interview, with a particular focus on the utility of this approach in child and adolescent psychiatry.

FINDING VALUE IN THE DIAGNOSTIC INTERVIEW

Given that most youth do not seek mental health treatment on their own, often their motivation to begin and remain in treatment resides largely with others, such as parents, teachers, or referral agencies.[3] Although this is a potential barrier toward building rapport with the young patient during the diagnostic interview, it is also important to consider that parents and caregivers can play a large role in these young patients' adherence to treatment. Thus, the child and adolescent clinician faces a high bar when it comes to the initial interview; developing rapport with the patient is not sufficient and must involve all of the caregivers present.

Diverse and vulnerable populations face particular barriers to receiving effective mental health care, including structural and logistical barriers related to such factors as health insurance and access to care, and sociocultural factors including stigma and mistrust in the mental health system.[4] Kerkorian and colleagues[5] found that parents were six times less likely to see the value of mental health treatment and to overcome structural barriers to care if they have felt disrespected by their child's mental health provider. In addition to impacting attrition rates, such perceptual barriers play a role in service underuse, especially among persons of color.[6,7] With these factors in mind, clinicians working with underserved populations may have particular reason to consider a strengths-based, positive approach to clinical assessment.

The positive approach to the diagnostic interview emphasizes respect and value toward each individual involved and may help provide a sense of hope to families who have experienced barriers to treatment including mistrust and fear, racism and discrimination, and differences in communication.[8] Additionally, when there are real or perceived sociodemographic differences between a clinician and patient, such as age, gender, race, sexual orientation, level of education, socioeconomic status, and so forth, the positive approach to the diagnostic interview may enhance rapport, because the clinician conveys an authentic desire to develop a holistic understanding of the child and family, rather than focus just on the chief complaint. Demonstrating an interest in what parents or family caregivers love most about the child, rather than getting right to the problem, shows a simultaneous respect for parents and caregivers and the roles they play in the child's life and for the child as a person beyond mental health diagnoses or behavioral labels. It may help to improve service utilization by families who need the support most, yet have experienced the biggest barriers.

WHY PRIME A PATIENT WITH POSITIVE EMOTIONS?

If a person is asked, "What is the opposite of heavy?" a fairly reasonable answer might be "light," as the variable is weight. If asked to name the opposite of sadness, "happiness" might be a common response, but this is actually misleading. Happiness and sadness are different feelings and developed for different reasons. In 1872, Charles Darwin published *Emotions in Man and Animals*, and highlighted a discussion that continues to be debated: why did humans evolve so many emotions? The negative emotions have been shown to have specific action tendencies: fear leads to the action of flight, anger to attack, and disgust can prevent the spread of disease or the ingestion of a toxin.[9] The original role of negative emotions was to keep humans alive; but the action tendencies of positive emotions are, as described by Fredrickson,[9] more often vague.[9] Functionally, love and lust can be specific in that they encourage reproduction, but many of the positive emotions such as joy, tranquility, and pride, do not lead to the immediate specific action tendencies as found in our negative emotions. Positive emotions are not the opposite of negative emotions; although negative emotions may have kept humans reactive and more likely to survive, the positive emotions have allowed humans to flourish.

Fredrickson developed the Broaden-and-Build Theory of Positive Emotions, a theoretic model for understanding how positive emotions have contributed to human evolution. Positive emotions most often "function as internal signals to *approach or continue*."[9] Positive emotions encourage "engagement in the environment" along with motivating people to pursue a thought or action.[9] Joy inspires people to be playful, creative, and encourages social and intellectual life. Interest, often activated by novelty, drives us to explore others and ourselves, whereas hope can help us generate "workable routes to desired goals," when confronted with challenge.[10(p258)] Gratitude, often considered the most prosocial emotion, encourages us to connect with those around us. Positive emotions do much more than make us feel good; they change the way we think and behave. Positive emotions encourage creativity, negotiation instead of withdrawal, and more "thorough, open-minded, flexible thinking and problem solving."[11(p528)] Priming is a technique in psychology where exposure to a stimulus influences the response to the next stimulus, or in this case, interaction. Primed with positive emotions, people's thought-action repertoires are broadened, and personal, physical, and intellectual resources grow.

The clinician who begins the interview focusing on negative emotions misses out on the opportunity to prime the patient with positive emotions. Asking about a patient's weakness, fear, anger, or sadness reveals the person's aversions to various circumstances in their world, yet may be another experience amplifying negative emotions and eliciting the desire to run away from the interview, withdraw from talking, or protest (as many child providers have experienced). Although the perception among mental health clinicians has always been that therapists can help patients by creating a safe place for the patient to talk about negative or painful emotions and experiences, this does not require that therapists speak with patients only about their negative emotions and experiences as they seek to cultivate resilience.

Linley has studied the way that people speak when discussing their strengths and their weaknesses. When describing weaknesses, Linley points out that people are more critical and unforgiving of themselves and they sound disengaged from the conversation, like they are holding something back.[12] In contrast, when people discuss their strengths the "sound and tone of their voice changes in pitch," they seem happy, and develop confidence.[12] When the clinician begins the interview focused on discovering what is right about the patient, pointing the flashlight on what makes the patient great, an opportunity emerges to elicit positive emotions in the patient. It is these positive emotions that create a therapeutic space filled with creativity, interest, novelty, and the desire to connect. This is the patient the clinician may have the most success with: someone who is open-minded, thinking flexibly, and ready to problem solve. In this emotional environment, the clinician can then pursue the challenges that are confronting the patient's well-being.

NOVELTY AND NEUROSCIENCE: HOW THE CLINICIAN CAN TAKE ADVANTAGE OF THE PATIENT'S REWARD CIRCUITS

Many people may have a preconception about receiving mental health treatment. For those who have never before sought treatment, some of these preconceptions may stem from the media's representation of psychotherapy in movies and television, and from societal stigma toward mental health disorders and views that individuals requiring mental health treatment are weak or inadequate. Additionally, many people do not seek mental health care simply because they do not believe it works.[13]

For those who have received treatment in the past, there might be an expectation of a rote clinical experience involving an intake highlighting their presenting problems, followed by sessions that target such problems or chief complaints. Past experiences that have not met an individual's expectations or may have been genuinely negative can result in resistance toward seeking support when needed or alternatively, showing up for treatment with a sense of skepticism. Such resistance can become an active process and a fundamental obstacle toward therapeutic progress.[14] Disbelief or negative attitudes toward treatment can interfere with a clinician's perceived efficacy and client motivation.[14] That said, although resistance was once considered nonadherence or a defense mechanism, it is natural to expect some ambivalence given that clients are expected to enter a relationship built on trust and intimacy and explore personal issues with someone they have just met for the first time.[14] Given that clients may be initially reluctant to engage in a process of discussing negative thoughts and emotions that can diminish self-efficacy and self-concept, the positive approach to the diagnostic interview may be a welcomed, unexpected, gratifying, and effective experience for patients.[14]

The positive diagnostic interview takes an innovative approach that is novel and unexpected to patients, and perhaps even to clinicians who have not considered this technique in their practice. Novelty, in general, has the tendency to engage individuals by capturing and maintaining attention while developing an interest into the experience.[15] Novel experiences can also be more satisfying to individuals than known experiences, and uncertainty can enhance positive experiences.[16] As such, the positive approach to the diagnostic interview can benefit clinician and patient. The approach has the potential to invigorate a clinician by exposing them to a new and exciting method for practice, and the patient is not only met by an enthusiastic and optimistic clinician but also an unforeseen pleasant experience that leaves them with a sense of hope and a desire for more.

Clinicians can capitalize on the neuroscience behind novelty to engage and retain patients and families in treatment. A novel, positive approach during the initial interview activates the hippocampus, which compares stimuli against existing memories, and the amygdala, which responds to emotional stimuli and strengthens associated long-term memories.[17] This neural activation supports the patient's preparedness, learning, and memory necessary for intended therapeutic change. The substantia nigra and ventral tegmental area, parts of the midbrain that respond to novel stimuli, are responsible for regulating motivation and reward. These neural processes not only prepare one's mental state for change but can also vitalize motivation in patients to engage in the novel experience. When patients anticipate a positive reward as a result of their engagement in treatment, the novel experience may result in a patient's genuine interest in a return visit. When working with children and families who are vulnerable to attrition before the completion of therapy, this approach may be an effective solution to improve treatment adherence.[18] Additionally, this approach has an inherent strength among adolescents who, developmentally, have a peaked sensitivity toward rewards.[19]

MANAGING RESISTANCES TO THE POSITIVE ASSESSMENT

All change is resisted—even good change. Any change, even a change for the better, is always accompanied by drawbacks and discomforts.
—Arnold Bennett

The clinician may encounter circumstances in which starting with the positive assessment is challenging. If there is an obviously negative affect in a family member, then it is best to address those feelings directly, validate them, and then outline how the concern behind the affect (the worry, the feeling of injustice, the frustrated attainment of a goal) will be addressed within the positive psychiatry interview structure. For example:

If you're like most parents who've waited so long to see me, my guess is that you're anxious to jump straight into describing your child's struggles. I want to reassure you now that we'll spend enough time on those struggles to understand them fully. We even know that hiding problems is developmentally appropriate for school-aged children, so we've had to develop ways of overcoming children's normal urge to keep their problems or difficulties private, and the positive assessment is the most effective method I've found.

Another more subtle but equally challenging situation is that of the overly compliant or people-pleasing family whose negative affect is less obvious. Clinicians who are optimistic, enthusiastic, and charismatic need to be mindful of their energy not resonating with the angst the family has been experiencing, and ending up with a false or skeptical acceptance to appease or please the exuberant interviewer, or to prevent themselves from being overwhelmed and feeling guilty for being more pessimistic. The clinician needs to deliberately focus on the family's affect at the beginning of the visit to look for more nuanced signs of underlying negative emotional states and underlying desires for validation that their distress and anguish are justified and that the patient is the cause of the family's problems. Otherwise, the positive assessment can be perceived as invalidating and overly protective of the clinician's feelings at the expense of the patient.

Another common situation is that of the distrusting or skeptical family. This distrust might be generally focused (eg, from trauma or experiences of persecutory racism[20]) or specific to mental health providers (eg, from previous invalidating experiences in treatment or hopelessness caused by lack of treatment efficacy). Such families often have the experience of not feeling known or seen by clinicians. Clinicians need to reassure the family that they will work hard to develop a holistic view of the family. For example:

It sounds like you've had some difficult experiences in the past that may have made trusting people seem pretty risky. I would like to earn your trust by getting to know each of you and your goals for coming here really well and by making my intentions really clear from the beginning. I'd first like to learn from you what you and your family look like when you're at your best and then learn from you what challenges you're facing that are getting in the way of you being at your best. What do you think about that plan? Are there any adjustments to the plan you think would be helpful?

Experienced mental health clinicians recognize in themselves certain feelings that tell them an assessment visit with a new family has been effective. After such interviews, clinicians typically feel connected with the family, engaged in their work, hopeful for the future, proud of the alliance they have built, and energized for the next opportunity to help a family in need. Without realizing it, clinicians are experiencing what Seligman calls PERMA, or the fundamental components of well-being in positive psychology: positive emotions, engagement, positive relationships, meaning, and accomplishment.[21]

The following section focuses on how clinicians can integrate positive and negative elements of a patient and family's experience via the PERMA model for well-being. Some might confuse this for a superficial "all is okay" approach, which focuses on the positive and minimizes the negative. To the contrary, it is precisely because this method elicits the positive within the interview that it enables the rapid development of a deeper sense of safety and trust, and allows patients to share the truly shameful, terrifying, and heartbreaking parts of their lives.

INTERVIEWING WITH PERMA IN MIND

The positive assessment is a powerful tool in the development of the therapeutic alliance, including the development of mutually agreed on treatment goals. In the positive assessment, the provider orients the family and patient to the session:

I'm going to start by learning how you feel and how you spend your time when you're at your best, as well as how you'd like to feel and spend your time in the near future. Having those images in our minds will help us figure out what success would look like at the end of all of your mental health treatment.

Most families tolerate this deviation from what they are expecting ("What is the problem that brings you here?"), although occasionally some families seek to ensure that their problems are identified early in the evaluation; in such cases, the clinician may need to hear their concerns or descriptions to acknowledge awareness of the problems first, and then shift to the positive interview format so that families do not become unnecessarily anxious or frustrated.

The provider can introduce the family to the PERMA model of mental well-being by describing each element. This process may be aided by writing the acronym down on a whiteboard or piece of paper that all in the room can see. At this point, some clinicians might also like to use Brown's "Circles Inside Squares" approach (**Fig. 1**) to visually orient the family to the fact that the clinician will also be asking about the most significant current barriers to mental well-being in addition to individual and environmental strengths and challenges.[22] Having this visual image often quells any rising anxiety in either caregivers or patient about whether or not significant problems (chief complaints) will be addressed.

Positive Emotions

The clinician then asks questions and makes supportive statements to encourage the sharing of things (eg, activities, events, cultural or religious practices, favorite foods)

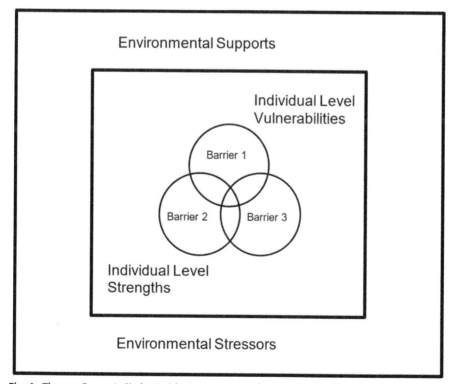

Fig. 1. Thomas Brown's Circles Inside Squares visual formulation method. (*Data from* Dweck CS. Mindset: the new psychology of success. New York: Random House; 2006.)

that bring the child and family positive emotions (see **Table 1** for example questions). While doing so, the clinicians monitor their own emotional tone and work diligently to stay attuned to the emotional tone of the family, recognizing that their reactions are heard best when they are "mirrored" and "marked," that is, when they accurately reflect the feelings of the family while also clearly remaining only reflections of their feelings and not the projected feelings of the clinician.[23]

This is not to say that the clinician should hide their genuine positive feelings. A well-executed positive assessment is fun, engaging, and meaningful for everyone involved. The important note is that just as a depressed provider's dysregulated response to a patient's sadness may damage the therapeutic alliance, the hyperexuberant clinician may overpower the patient's feelings or get them so charged up that they lose their narrative capacity.

Engagement

Once a thorough inventory of what brings the youth and family positive emotions has been completed, then the clinician encourages them to describe activities of engagement. These are the physical activities or hobbies that immerse them in the present moment, creating a sense of absorption in the process (**Table 1** provides example clinician questions). These experiences leave people feeling invigorated and are often described as being challenging and interesting. Of note, engagement can occur alone or in a group setting, so clinicians should ask about experiences across settings. As when discussing positive emotions, the clinician is well-served by appropriately connecting to the patient's experience of engagement. The clinician may point out that meeting a family for the first time is an example of an engaging activity for themselves.

Relationships

This next section of the interview is familiar to most clinicians. However, instead of focusing on the number of friendships and whether the youth has a best friend, the positive assessment of relationships is most interested in the quality and the youth's level of satisfaction. To get at the quality of relationships, the clinician likely needs to elicit the perspectives of the youth and the caregivers. The interviewer must also be aware of applying their own implicit biases (eg, that a female patient will more likely prefer artistic/musical activities to meet friends than sports) or judgments about the quality of the youth's relationships, while also not missing opportunities to empathize with a lonely or socially disconnected child or adolescent.

This is also a valuable opportunity to learn about the youth's aspirations for their relationships. Although they may not have the relationships they want in their life currently, they may have a clear picture of what kind of relationships they would like to have in the future. Sometimes youth may be able to describe that they seek relationships like those described by or observed in others they may know (eg, real people they observe or celebrities they admire). Clarifying that image moves the patient and the provider closer to relationship-oriented goals for treatment.

Meaning

Man's search for meaning is a primary force in his life and not a 'secondary rationalization' of instinctual drives. This meaning is unique and specific in that it must and can be fulfilled by him alone; only then does it achieve a significance which will satisfy his own will to meaning.
                                                    —*Victor E. Frankl, Man's Search for Meaning*[24]

Table 1
PERMA interview questions

PERMA Element	Interview Questions
Positive emotions	**Caregiver(s)** What makes ____ happy? Excited? Joyful? Calm? **Child** Can you describe how you feel when you are totally calm? What helps calm you? Think of a time you felt great joy—what makes you feel joy? **Adolescent** What do you do for fun? What makes you happy?
Engagement	**Caregiver(s)** What does ___ do for hours? What does ___ do where they just lose themselves into it and may even forget about time? What does _____ "persist" at? **Child** What are you interested in? What do you like to think about? What do you most like to do? What could you do all day long and never get bored? **Adolescent** What do you lose yourself in doing? What do get so interested in that you lose all track of time? What do you stay with or "persist" at?
Relationships	**Caregiver(s)** What are ___'s friendships/relationships like? What does _____ do well with others? With family members? **Young Child** Who do you like to play with? What nice things do they say about you? Who do you like to talk to about fun things that happen to you? **School-Aged Child** What good things do others say about you? What makes you a good friend? Who are you a good friend to? How did you make your good friends? **Adolescent** Are you happy with the friends that you have? Who do you really get along with in your family? What do you like about that relationship? Who do you admire? Who do you have the most respect for?
Meaning	**Caregiver(s)** What does ____ value/care about? What purpose or meaning do you find in parenting? **Child** What makes you feel important? Do you have any opportunities to help other people? How do you feel when you are helpful? **Adolescent** What matters most to you? Have your values changed over time? How so?
Accomplishments	**Caregiver(s)** What makes ____ feel good about themselves? What makes you proud of ___? **Child** What do you feel like you are good at? What have you worked hard at and felt successful about?

(continued on next page)

Table 1 (continued)

PERMA Element	Interview Questions
	Adolescent
	What things have you done that you think you'll remember with a smile when you're older?
	What would you and others say you are your biggest accomplishments?

As Frankl eloquently states, individuals have their own unique meaning to fulfill. As clinicians, our responsibility is to help our patients elucidate that meaning so that we can help them move back onto the path toward leading a purposeful life. Even though most young children cannot yet understand the abstract concept of "meaning" per se, they can clearly state what is important to them, what they care about, and what they look forward to. The adolescent may be able to expand on this by explaining what they value, what they think others should value, and what brings them a sense of peace. Even young children are aware of how they spend their hours, which is a useful measure of what they find most meaningful. How they spend their hours is sometimes inconsistent with what they say they care about. For example, some may say they most value being a good friend, yet spend much more of their time alone working on resume-building projects in the pursuit of admission to a competitive college.

Meaning is also helpful to discuss with caregivers. For many caregivers, much of their purpose is directed toward promoting their child's well-being and they may feel thwarted in their efforts to create a happy life for their child. Caregivers' sense of meaning is disrupted when they recognize undesirable outcomes in their children. These discussions provide valuable opportunities to elicit caregiver emotions, positive and negative, around the experience of trying to maintain that sense of meaning in the face of adversity. When the caregiver feels that the provider understands what is meaningful to them, a trust emerges that the clinician will be able to reconnect them with the purpose that drives so much of their behavior. This is also a wonderful opportunity for clinicians to join and connect with caregivers by noting that promoting the well-being of youth is also central to meaning in their own life.

Accomplishments

For many children presenting for youth mental health treatment, the feelings of having failed or having disappointed themselves or others are all too familiar. Youth who are struggling functionally typically receive a significant amount of well-meaning negative feedback from caregivers, teachers, peers, and themselves. Youth often struggle to view this feedback in the context of their strengths; instead, they spend much of their time either acutely feeling shame, ready to lash out or shut down at the mere hint of criticism from others. Unfortunately, shame elicits feelings of inferiority and worthlessness typically resulting in attempts to hide or disappear.[25] Eliciting shame at the outset of the initial interview impedes forming a connection with the identified patient and gathering valuable information from them.

In this section of the interview, the clinician is trying to evoke the feeling of authentic pride, which "arises from a positive evaluation of one's specific achievements ('I did that well'), whereas hubristic pride is evoked when the person perceives the achievement as a product of the great self ('I did that well')."[26] The clinician asks about things the youth has accomplished that bring about feelings of success, value, authentic pride, and/or achievement.

CONSOLIDATION OF ALLIANCE AND TRANSITION TO PSYCHIATRIC REVIEW OF SYSTEMS

Once the clinician and family have collaboratively constructed a picture of the patient at the optimal state of well-being, then the clinician proceeds to summarizing the findings, checking with the family to see if anything is missing, and transitioning into a discussion of obstacles getting in the way of the patient's well-being. The framing of these barriers is important because the goal is to maintain the sense of hope and trust that developed through the PERMA assessment. When discussing challenges, as opposed to the traditional assessment's use of "problem" or "complaint," the patient retains an internal locus of control and challenges can be overcome and serve as a stimulus for growth.

Greene and Ablon[27] described a framework for approaching psychological barriers for children with the phrase "kids do well if they can" as opposed to "kids do well if they want to." In their work, they adjusted this message to further include the adults in a child's life: "People are doing the best they can with what they've got." They described psychological challenges as "lagging skills" and outline the "thinking skill" domains of executive functioning, language-processing, emotion regulation, cognitive flexibility, and social skills.[27]

In this model, parents are asked to rate the individual skills in each skill domain on a Likert scale from "consistent strength" to "consistent difficulty." Treatment plans then focus on building up lagging skills in identified areas of difficulty. This may sound familiar for clinicians familiar with Dweck's[27] "growth mindset," which highlights that one's abilities are not static. Skills are developed and individuals grow if they put in effort, receive effective coaching, and persist through continued practice. Discussing psychological and environmental challenges this way allows the clinician and family to focus on building resilience in the child and family as opposed to fixing (specific) problems. This also allows for a richer discussion of how the identified symptoms are functionally interfering with the youth's mental well-being.

This naturally leads into the final step of establishing the therapeutic alliance: collaboratively developing and agreeing on treatment methods aimed at helping the youth and family overcome the described obstacles to mental well-being and using the family's internal and environmental strengths. The positive assessment approach helps the clinician and family keep the collaboratively developed image of the flourishing patient as a guiding light from assessment through treatment. By eliciting the hopes and desires of a patient, and uncovering the barriers they face toward achieving them, patient-centered treatment goals are clearly outlined and ready to be collaboratively shaped by clinician input. Once the team agrees on goals, the clinician then works together with the family to decide which treatment methods are the best fit for reaching those goals. This is a unique opportunity for a deliberate infusion of hope through the clinician's affirmation that the treatment plan will be helpful. At the conclusion of the interview (or earlier), the clinician may support the alliance by congratulating the youth and caregivers, as appropriate, for their bravery, noting that it takes a tremendous amount of courage to seek help and to share one's strengths and challenges.

SUMMARY

The positive assessment accomplishes a few goals simultaneously:

1. It deliberately primes the session with positive emotions, which encourages the patient to think more flexibly, trust the clinician, and enhance rapport.
2. It incorporates a history of the patient's well-being.

3. It elevates the establishment of treatment goals at the outset of the interview.

Child mental health clinicians have always used humor, games, and general "goofiness" to prime patients with positive emotions.[28] The positive assessment prioritizes the need to positively prime patients while also developing an often-neglected component of the patient's history: their PERMA. The positive interview can improve all clinicians' clinical interviews by creating better rapport leading to more accurate diagnoses and more effective treatment plans. Such treatment plans may create more than amelioration of suffering, by cultivating each patient's awareness and practices for well-being.

ACKNOWLEDGMENTS

The authors acknowledge Jeffrey Bostic, MD, for his significant contributions to developing the questions in **Table 1**.

REFERENCES

1. Huntington B, Kuhn N. Communication gaffes: a root cause of malpractice claims. Proc (Bayl Univ Med Cent) 2003;16(2):157–61 [discussion: 161].
2. Lambert MJ. Implications of outcome research for psychotherapy integration. In: Nor cross JC, Goldfried MR, editors. Handbook of psychotherapy integration. New York: Basic Books; 1992. p. 94–129.
3. de Haan AM, Boon AE, de Jong JTVM, et al. A review of mental health treatment dropout by ethnic minority youth. Transcult Psychiatry 2018;55(1):3–30.
4. Acri MC, Bornheimer LA, O'Brien K, et al. A model of integrated health care in a poverty-impacted community in New York City: importance of early detection and addressing potential barriers to intervention implementation. Soc Work Health Care 2016;55(4):314–27.
5. Kerkorian D, McKay M, Bannon WM Jr. Seeking help a second time: parents'/caregivers' characterizations of previous experiences with mental health services for their children and perceptions of barriers to future use. Am J Orthopsychiatry 2006;76(2):161–6.
6. Alegria M, Atkins M, Farmer E, et al. One size does not fit all: taking diversity, culture and context seriously. Adm Policy Ment Health 2010;37(1–2):48–60.
7. Godoy L, Carter AS. Identifying and addressing mental health risks and problems in primary care pediatric settings: a model to promote developmental and cultural competence. Am J Orthopsychiatry 2013;83(1):73–88.
8. U.S. Public Health Service. U.S. Public Health Service. Mental health: culture race and ethnicity. A supplement to mental health: a report of the surgeon general. Available at: http://www.ct.gov/dmhas/lib/dmhas/publications/mhethnicity.pdf. Accessed August 14, 2018.
9. Fredrickson BL. The role of positive emotions in positive psychology: the broaden-and-build theory of positive emotions. Am Psychol 2001;56(3):218–26.
10. Snyder CR, Rand KL, Sigmon DR. Hope theory: a member of the positive psychology family. In: Snyder CR, Lopez SJ, editors. Handbook of positive psychology. New York: Oxford University Press; 2001. p. 257–76.
11. Isen AM. A role for neuropsychology in understanding the facilitating influence of positive affect on social behavior and cognitive processes. In: Snyder CR, Lopez SJ, editors. Handbook of positive psychology. New York: Oxford University Press; 2001. p. 528–40.

12. Linley A. Average to A+: realising strengths in yourself and others. Coventry (England): Capp Press; 2008. p. 72–111.
13. Anker MG, Duncan BL, Sparks JA. Using client feedback to improve couple therapy outcomes: a randomized clinical trial in a naturalistic setting. J Consult Clin Psychol 2009;77(4):693–704.
14. Watson JC. Addressing client resistance: recognizing and processing in-Session occurrences. In: VISTAS online. 2006. Available at: https://www.counseling.org/Resources/Library/VISTAS/vistas06_online-only/Watson.pdf. Accessed August 10, 2018.
15. Bunzeck N, Düzel E. Absolute coding of stimulus novelty in the human substantia nigra/VTA. Neuron 2006;51(3):369–79.
16. Lyubomirsky S. New love: a short shelf life. New York Times 2012;SR1.
17. Cooper B. Why getting new things makes us feel so good: novelty and th brain 2018. Available at: https://blog.bufferapp.com/novelty-and-the-brain-how-to-learn-more-and-improve-your-memory.
18. Ingoldsby EM. Review of interventions to improve family engagement and retention in parent and child mental health programs. J Child Fam Stud 2010;19(5): 629–45.
19. Casey BJ, Jones RM. Neurobiology of the adolescent brain and behavior: implications for substance use disorders. J Am Acad Child Adolesc Psychiatry 2010; 49(12):1189–201 [quiz: 1285].
20. Hagiwara N, Dovidio JF, Eggly S, et al. The effects of racial attitudes on affect and engagement in racially discordant medical interactions between non-Black physicians and Black patients. Group Process Intergroup Relat 2016;19(4):509–27.
21. Seligman MEP. Flourish: a visionary new understanding of happiness and well-being. New York: Simon and Schuster; 2012.
22. Brown TE. Circles inside squares: a graphic organizer to focus diagnostic formulations. J Am Acad Child Adolesc Psychiatry 2005;44(12):1309–12.
23. Fonagy P. Affect regulation, mentalization, and the development of the self. New York: Other Press, LLC; 2002.
24. Frankl VE, Kushner HS, Winslade WJ. Man's search for meaning. Boston: Beacon Press; 2006.
25. Muris P, Meesters C. Small or big in the eyes of the other: on the developmental psychopathology of self-conscious emotions as shame, guilt, and pride. Clin Child Fam Psychol Rev 2013;17(1):19–40.
26. Greene RW, Stuart Ablon J. Treating explosive kids: the collaborative problem-solving approach. New York: Guilford Press; 2005.
27. Dweck CS. Mindset: the new psychology of success. New York: Random House; 2006.
28. Drell MJ. My use of humor in therapy: a performance-in-practice self-study. J Am Acad Child Adolesc Psychiatry 2015;54(3):159–61.

Promoting Mental Health and Wellness in Youth Through Physical Activity, Nutrition, and Sleep

Daniel K. Hosker, MD[a],*, R. Meredith Elkins, PhD[b,c,1],
Mona P. Potter, MD[c,d,1]

KEYWORDS

- Mental health • Wellness • Exercise • Sports • Nutrition • Diet • Sleep
- Child and adolescent

KEY POINTS

- From 3 to 5 days of moderate to vigorous aerobic exercise for 45 to 60 minutes confers benefits to youth physical and mental wellness. Additional benefits are seen with sports participation.
- Nutritional patterns that are high in a variety of fruits and vegetables, whole grains, seafood, and nuts, moderate in low-fat dairy products, low in red meat, and very limited in processed foods, saturated and trans fats, added sugars, and sodium have been associated with improved mental health outcomes across the lifespan.
- Following age-appropriate recommendations for sleep duration is associated with improvements in mental health and well-being. Engaging in consistent and calming bedtime routines, creating a restful and comforting sleep environment, and ensuring that children's physical and emotional needs are met during the daytime can increase the likelihood of obtaining adequate sleep duration.
- Seligman's PERMA (positive emotions, engagement, relationships, meaning, and accomplishment) model is a useful construct to approach improving physical activity, eating, and sleep to yield improved physical and mental wellness in youth.

Disclosures: None.
[a] Psychiatry, Massachusetts General Hospital, 32 Fruit St, Boston, MA 02114, USA; [b] McLean Anxiety Mastery Program, McLean Hospital, 799 Concord Avenue, Cambridge, MA 02138, USA; [c] Department of Psychiatry, Harvard Medical School, 25 Shattuck St, Cambridge, MA 02115, USA; [d] McLean Child and Adolescent Psychiatry Outpatient Services, McLean Hospital, 115 Mill St, Belmont, MA 02478, USA
[1] Present address: 799 Concord Avenue, Cambridge MA 02138.
* Corresponding author. 4 Emerson Place Apartment 1113, Boston, MA 02114.
E-mail address: dhosker@mgh.harvard.edu

Child Adolesc Psychiatric Clin N Am 28 (2019) 171–193
https://doi.org/10.1016/j.chc.2018.11.010
1056-4993/19/© 2018 Elsevier Inc. All rights reserved.

childpsych.theclinics.com

INTRODUCTION

Approximately 1 in every 4 to 5 youth in the United States meet criteria for a mental disorder with severe impairment before they reach adulthood.[1] Improving health care and implementing practices to decrease vulnerability to psychiatric symptoms is a vital part of treatment of this population. Conventional first-line treatments such as cognitive behavior therapy (CBT) and psychopharmacology may be moderately effective, but too often fail to improve some symptoms, with medications carrying a risk for serious side effects.[2,3] Alternative or augmenting treatment interventions such as incorporating physical activity, improving nutrition, and optimizing sleep allow clinicians to fashion a more comprehensive approach to mental health treatment of youth.

The landscape of youth mental health and wellness is evolving as providers increasingly view interventions through a more holistic lens. Although many research studies have shown the benefits of physical activity, nutrition, and sleep in youth, few studies show how these factors interact with emotional health and wellness. The existing research in this area is largely cross-sectional, which precludes a demonstration of causality, and is also limited by researchers' use of heterogeneous protocols and measurements, small sample sizes, and nonclinical participants. These methodological limitations highlight the complexity involved with researching such dynamic variables and interactions. Given the lack of a robust evidence base, it is difficult to standardize recommendations, particularly in relation to physical activity and nutrition. However, the existing research studies suggest that optimizing physical activity, nutrition, and sleep confers numerous benefits for youth mental health and wellness, and exerts a positive impact on the developmental trajectory of young people vulnerable to, or struggling with, psychiatric disorders.

PHYSICAL ACTIVITY AND SPORTS
Clinical Relevance and Current Research

A significant body of research shows that being more physically active has significant benefits for everyone, regardless of age, sex, race, ethnicity, or current fitness level.[4] The US Department of Health and Human Services recommends that preschool-aged children (ages 3–5 years) be physically active throughout the day to enhance growth and development, and children and adolescents aged 6 to 17 years should engage in 60 minutes or more of physical activity each day (with 3 days a week including muscle- strengthening and bone-strengthening each), with most of the 60 minutes being of moderate-intensity or vigorous-intensity aerobic physical activity, to enhance physical wellness.[4] Although this level of physical activity yields improved cardiorespiratory and muscular fitness, stronger bones, healthier metabolic biomarkers, and more favorable body composition, only 20% of US high school students meet these guidelines.[4] A growing body of literature suggests that physical activity also yields mental health and wellness benefits, although precise recommendations for type, amount, and frequency remain elusive.

There are small to moderate positive associations between physical activity and positive mental health traits, including social-emotional and academic functioning in youth, as summarized in **Table 1**.

Similarly, improving physical activity can also confer benefits to youth at risk for, or with, certain psychiatric symptoms and disorders, as summarized in **Table 2**.

Participation in organized and/or competitive sports offers a unique gateway to physical activity. Children can engage in sports either as an individual or as a member of a team, although individual sports have been found to yield fewer psychological

Table 1
Associations between physical activity and social-emotional and academic wellness and possible clinical implications

Domain of Benefits	Trait	Clinical Implications
Social-Emotional	• Enhanced self-concept[a,5] • Increased life skills[a,5] • Improved self-esteem[a,5] • Protective for shy children[a,b,5]	• Improved self-perception and value of own qualities and abilities • More likely to express confidence in self • Increased engagement in novel activities and/or new situations • By learning to tolerate distress, can challenge self further, and reap benefits when overcoming new tasks
Academic	• Improved classroom behavior, with decreased disruptive behaviors[6] • Improved academic achievement[6] • Cognitive and metacognitive benefits including learning, memory, attention management, and processing speed[4,7–9]	• Improvements in grades and test scores[6] • Reduce the likelihood of negative classroom behaviors[6] • Greater confidence in school-based tasks • Improved ability to attend to academic and daily tasks (eg, homework, quizzes, tests)[6]

[a] Associations seen with sports participation.
[b] As measured by decreased reports of anxiety symptoms.

benefits, and significantly fewer social benefits than team participation.[5] Children who are active in sports are more likely to be physically active in adulthood, which is critically important because more physically active adults lead physically and emotionally healthier lives.[5,23]

How It Works

The mechanisms of action by which physical activity and sports confer benefits to different domains of mental health and wellness are multifactorial, but they tend to be in 2 broad categories: neurobiological and psychosocial. Although the neurobiological cannot be separated from the psychosocial, and vice versa, conceptualizing it in this way can be helpful, as summarized in **Table 3**.

Clinical Assessment

Before recommending physical activity or sports as part of a therapeutic intervention, it is important to clarify what the child is already doing, the child's activity preferences, and potential obstacles to being physically active. The answers to these questions may prompt further inquiry if, for example, the clinician suspects that the child is exercising too much in the context of an eating disorder or too little because of ongoing medical issues. Sample questions to help in the assessment of children's physical activity are listed in **Table 4**. It is important to ask these of the parent and child if possible, because there can be discrepancies that are important to address. These questions can be modified to be asked directly of the child as the clinical context allows.

Recommendations for Physical Activity

Clinicians should consider prescribing physical activity as a way of promoting both physical and emotional health in youth, especially given the increasing evidence

Table 2
Associations between physical activity and psychiatric disorders

Depression and suicidality	• Protective effect against depression across age, gender, and geographic regions across the world[10] • Treatment effect sizes similar to that of antidepressant and CBT therapy for depressive symptoms in children and adolescents[2,11–13] • Lower odds of sadness, suicidal ideation, or suicidal attempts in high school students[a,14] • Reduction in suicidal ideation and attempts in bullied high school students[a,15] • Decreased suicidal ideation and intention in adolescents involved with team sports[b,g] • Decreased hopelessness, depression, and suicidality among college students[16] • Inverse bidirectional association between depressive symptoms and physical activity (ie, increased physical activity precedes decreased depressive symptoms, and increased depressive symptoms precede decreased physical activity)[17]
ADHD	• Improvements in core ADHD symptoms (inattention, hyperactivity, and impulsivity)[c,3] • Improved social, motor, behavioral, and emotional functioning[d,18] • Physical activity in adolescence may decrease ADHD symptoms in early adulthood[19]
Anxiety	• May improve symptoms of anxiety in children and adolescents[6] • Decreased social anxiety with lowered social isolation[5,g]
Substance use	• Lower levels of alcohol, cigarette, and marijuana use among high school students[e,20]
Psychosis and antipsychotic use	• Decreased physical activity and poorer cardiorespiratory fitness have been seen in adolescents who develop a psychotic illness[21] • Lower measures of adiposity and improved insulin resistance in children treated with a second-generation antipsychotic[f,22]

Abbreviation: ADHD, attention-deficit/hyperactivity disorder.
 [a] In high school students who exercised 4 to 5 d/wk compared with those who exercised 0 to 1 d/wk.
 [b] Benefits were lost when they discontinued playing sports.
 [c] Effects seen primarily with aerobic exercise.
 [d] Effects seen in medicated and unmedicated children with ADHD.
 [e] Although team sports were associated with higher levels of alcohol and smokeless tobacco use, physical activity mitigated some of the effects between team sports and alcohol use. Physical activity and being on a team were both shown to decrease cigarette and marijuana use.[20]
 [f] Seen in children who met a minimal recommendation for daily physical activity compared with those who did not.
 [g] Associations seen with sports participation.

regarding the negative health impact of sedentary behaviors, with US children spending approximately 7.7 h/d (55% of their monitored waking time) being sedentary.[4]

As discussed earlier, it is difficult to draw conclusions regarding optimal types or "doses" of physical activity for mental health benefits given the overall heterogeneous nature of the research and lack of methodologically rigorous studies. However, common trends among the data across mental health and wellness domains suggest that to obtain the mental health benefits, physical activity in youth should involve:

• At least 45 to 60 minutes of physical activity each day[2,4,10,14,18]
• From 3 to 5 days a week of moderate to vigorous aerobic activity[2,4,10,14,18]

Table 3
Means by which physical activity and sports may confer benefits to youth mental wellness

Conceptual System	Mechanism of Action
Neurobiological	• Modify inflammatory and oxidative stress responses[10] • Promote neurogenesis, synaptogenesis, myelination, and angiogenesis to aid brain development through neurotrophic factors (such as BDNF)[2,3,10,24] • Modulate monoamines (serotonin, dopamine, norepinephrine), endorphins, and endocannabinoids[2,3,10,24] • HPA axis regulation[2]
Psychosocial	• Behavioral activation with positive reinforcement[2] • Satisfy basic psychological needs for social connectedness and autonomy[24] • Mastery of a skillset[2,24] • Promote confidence through achievement[2,24] • Exposure to difficult situations and using distress tolerance • Increasing overall self-efficacy and self-concept[2]

Abbreviations: BDNF, brain-derived neurotropic factor; HPA, hypothalamic-pituitary-adrenal.

Table 4
Example questions of parents when assessing physical activity in youth in the context of a mental health evaluation

	Example Questions
Type	• What types of activities or sports does your child participate in? • Are these activities mostly aerobic (eg, running, swimming, soccer) or anaerobic (eg, push-ups/sit-ups, weight lifting, tug-of-war)?
Frequency	• How many days in a week does your child exercise or play sports? • What does your child do during "spare time"? • How consistently is the child exercising or staying physically active? (eg, spurts every so often, only during a sports season)
Duration	• How many minutes does your child exercise on average each day/week? • Do you have any worries that your child exercises too much? If yes, why do you think so?
Intensity	• When your child is exercising or playing sports, is the intensity most comparable with walking, jogging, or running? • Does your child usually end up sweating? • Is your child breathing hard during some, most, or all of the activity?
Preferred exercise	• What is your child's favorite way to be physically active? • Does your child prefer to play sports alone or on a team? • What have you seen your child enjoy most while engaged in physical activity?
Obstacles to physical activity	• Is there anything keeping your child from being more physically active? • Are there any medical concerns regarding your child being more physically active? • Does your child have appropriate strength and motor coordination? • Any concerns for bullying when your child is playing/practicing physical activities? • What other activities compete with time for physical activities? (eg, screen time, hanging out)
Supporting questions	• How has physical activity altered your child's nutrition? • How has physical activity affected your child's sleep? • Do you believe that your child is able to appropriately recover from the physical activity?

- Understanding that it might take at least 8 weeks of engagement before recognizing most benefits, although short-term benefits may be seen after as little as 1 bout of physical activity[2,4,10,14,18]

Fortunately, these guidelines align with the physical activity recommendations for youth from the US Department of Health and Human Services. **Table 5** summarizes clinical considerations when increasing physical activity and selecting appropriate activities for youth, adopted from the US Department of Health and Human Services' Physical Activity Guidelines for Americans, 2nd edition.[4]

The most important role a provider can play is to guide the exploration for an appropriate and enjoyable physical activity for a child, especially in younger children, in whom physical activity can be introduced as "play," and establishing an active lifestyle may yield benefits throughout a lifetime. Similarly, encouraging a child's participation in organized sports can be helpful in the right context, and may provide mental health benefits beyond increased physical activity alone. By fostering a best-fit activity, clinicians can yield improved compliance in the subset of youth who may otherwise have ambivalence or disinterest preventing them from participating. To further address ambivalence regarding participation, clinicians can use motivational interviewing techniques focusing on the goals, values, and interests of the child.

NUTRITION SCIENCE
Clinical Relevance and Current Research

A global obesity epidemic (United States currently ranked #1 in childhood obesity rates [12.7%]) has called attention to the need for intervention in multiple domains, including diet and nutrition.[25] Emerging evidence argues the case for nutritional awareness not only for its effects on physical health, but also because of its relationship with mental health and well-being. Much of the investigation historically has focused on the role of individual nutrients on mental health. For example, magnesium,[26] zinc,[27] and omega-3 fatty acids[28] have been studied in relation to anxiety and depression.

However, recent focus has broadened the scope to considering dietary patterns. Data that support an association between unhealthy patterns of eating and poor mental health (eg, depression, anxiety), as well as healthy patterns of eating and improved mental health, are emerging for all stages of life. **Table 6** summarizes major findings, including 1 adult randomized control trial, the Supporting the Modification of lifestyle In Lowered Emotional States (SMILES) trial.[41]

How It Works

Multiple pathways have been proposed in the association between diet and mental health, including (but not limited to) inflammation,[42] oxidative stress,[43] and changes in brain structure.[44] For example, unhealthy diet patterns have been associated with lower left hippocampal volume in animal and human studies, as well as the reverse for adults with healthy diet patterns, possibly mediated via brain-derived neurotropic factor.[29,45]

In addition, although in early stages, there has been growing interest in the gut microbiome (the approximately 100 trillion microorganisms that exist in the gastrointestinal tract) and its relationship with mental health.[46] The gut microbiome has been noted to be a virtual organ, producing metabolites that influence the host in many ways, with emerging evidence showing cross-influence with multiple systems, including neurobehavioral, metabolic, immune, and endocrine systems.[47] Although most data regarding the microbiota gut-brain connection currently come from animal models, human studies are emerging.[46,48,49]

Table 5
Clinical considerations when increasing and selecting physical activities for youth

	Clinical Consideration	Clinical Example/Recommendations
Increasing Physical Activity	Start early	• Encourage play at home and in the neighborhood • Provide time for structured and unstructured physical activity in and out of school • Promote activities the child can enjoy for a lifetime (eg, swimming, cycling)
	Start low, go slow	• Risk of injury is directly related to the gap between usual level of activity and a new level of activity. Keep the gap small, allowing the body to adapt • Use the child's level of fitness to guide the level of effort expected • First, increase the number of minutes (duration) of an activity, then the number of days (frequency), then increase from moderate to vigorous intensity • Can add light-intensity to moderate-intensity activities (eg, short walk) to weekly routine • Increase activity by small amounts every week or two for youth (considering age, level of fitness, and level of experience) • Keep activities enjoyable • Vary activities to avoid muscle overuse injuries
	Medical clearance	• Although medical clearance should not be necessary for most children, periodic monitoring and collaboration with relevant providers may be appropriate for children with known medical conditions that may be adversely affected by rigorous exercise[3,4]
	Replace sedentary behavior with activity when possible	• Replace TV watching after school with sports participation • Encourage walking or biking when possible instead of driving • Limit and replace screen time with family activities and outside games

Choosing a Physical Activity by Age and Aerobic Intensity[a]	Preschool-aged children	• Moderate intensity
		  ○ Tag, playing on playground, riding a tricycle or bicycle; games requiring catching, throwing, or kicking
		• Vigorous intensity
		  ○ Running, skipping, dancing, jumping, gymnastics, swimming

	School-aged children	• Moderate intensity
		  ○ Brisk walking, riding a bicycle, hiking, swimming, games that require catching and throwing
		• Vigorous intensity
		  ○ Running, riding a bicycle, jumping rope, cross-country skiing, sports (eg, soccer, basketball, tennis)

	Adolescents	• Moderate intensity
		  ○ Brisk walking, riding a bicycle, recreational activities (eg, kayaking, hiking, swimming)
		• Vigorous intensity
		  ○ Running, riding a bicycle, martial arts, vigorous dancing, sports (eg, soccer, basketball, tennis)

(continued on next page)

	Clinical Consideration	Clinical Example/Recommendations
Table 5 (continued)		
Special Considerations	During the transition to adolescence, physical activity in girls decreases significantly compared with boys (this disparity persists into adulthood)	• Female youth may need additional support and encouragement to maintain beneficial levels of physical activity • This may be provided by health professionals, parents, coaches, teachers, peers, and so forth
	Children and adolescents with disabilities are more likely to be inactive than those without disabilities	• Youth with disabilities should partner with a health care or physical activity professional to understand appropriate types and amounts of physical activity for them to assist in decreasing inactivity

[a] Because the evidence for mental health and wellness benefits in youth are most supported from aerobic activities, these are presented here.

Adapted from US Department of Health and Human Services. Physical activity guidelines for Americans. 2nd edition. Washington, DC: US Department of Health and Human Services; 2018.

Although there is a heritable component to people's microbiota compositions, environmental factors such as diet, stress, and medications are thought to have a larger influence.[47,50,51] Animal models have shown that an anxious phenotype can be transferred via gut microbiota, and manipulation of the gut microbiota (eg, with probiotics or antibiotics) can influence depression-like behaviors.[49]

Application of knowledge of the gut-brain relationship is a work in progress. Diversity of gut microbiota (rather than the concentration of any particular microorganism species) seems to be an indicator of a healthy gut.[47] Probiotics are marketed for their possible role in increasing "good bacteria," and therefore potentially benefitting mental health; however, the role of particular microbiota has yet to be fully elucidated, leaving many questions about the particular application of probiotics in the treatment of mental health problems.[47,48]

Clinical Assessment

Many factors contribute to food choice, including (but not limited to) biological need/appetite, taste preference/sensory stimulation, family/peer/social/cultural influence, habit/routine, cost/access/availability, mood/emotions/craving, health attitudes, and weight awareness. Given the impact on physical and mental health, clinicians are encouraged to evaluate for food insecurity (lack of consistent access to adequate food). The who, what, when, why, and where of eating patterns can offer opportunities to recognize processes that are going well and help bring attention to areas in need of intervention. Given the potential impact of the family system on the eating patterns of children, thorough assessment incorporates nutritional patterns of the family system.[52] Sample questions and associated recommendations for parents are listed in **Table 7** to assist in this assessment. These questions can be modified to be asked directly of the child as the clinical context allows.

Table 6
Association between dietary pattern and mental/emotional health across the life span

Stage of Life	Mental Health Outcomes
Prenatal and early life	• High adherence to unhealthy diet during pregnancy associated with increased risk of child externalizing problems[29–31] • Children with high level of unhealthy diet or low level of healthy diet postnatally had higher levels of both internalizing and externalizing problems by 5 y old[32]

Childhood and adolescence	• A review of 20 studies across 11 countries found support for an association between unhealthy diet and increased odds of mental health difficulties and between healthy dietary patterns and better mental health[33]
	Prospective studies:
	• Jacka and colleagues,[34] 2011: a study of nearly 3000 Australian adolescents, predominantly from higher socioeconomic backgrounds
	  ○ Better diet quality at baseline predicted better mental health at follow-up even after adjustment for mental health at baseline
	  ○ Improvements in diet quality were associated with improved mental health score at 2-year follow-up, whereas reductions in diet quality were associated with declining psychological functioning
	  ○ Mental health at baseline did not predict diet quality at 2-year follow-up
	• McMartin and colleagues,[35] 2012: 3757 fifth graders in Nova Scotia participated as part of the Children's Lifestyle and School performance Study (CLASS) survey
	  ○ Diet quality was not significantly associated with visits to a health care provider for internalizing disorder
	  ○ Dietary variety may reduce the risk of developing internalizing disorders
	  ○ One-third of children with the highest fish consumption had lower rates of being diagnosed with internalizing disorder
	• Jacka and colleagues,[36] 2013: evaluated >2000 students from ethnically diverse and socially deprived backgrounds and included a wide range of potentially confounding variables
	  ○ Cross-sectional study found an association between unhealthy diet and mental health difficulties
	  ○ Prospective study found that unhealthy and healthy diet scores did not significantly predict mental health status at 3-year follow-up, although patterns of associations were in the same direction as the cross-sectional analysis
	• Trapp and colleagues,[37] 2016: 746 adolescents participated as part of the Western Australian Pregnancy Cohort (Raine) Study
	  ○ Western (unhealthy) dietary pattern at 14 y old was positively associated with greater externalizing behaviors at 17 y old in girls
	  ○ No other statistically significant associations were observed after full adjustment of confounders
	• Winpenny and colleagues,[38] 2018: 603 adolescents participated as part of the ROOTS study (United Kingdom), participants were from higher socioeconomic status categories, adjustments made for sociodemographic, anthropometric, behavioral, and psychological factors in longitudinal analysis
	  ○ There were no prospective associations between healthy diet at 14 y of age and depressive symptoms at 17 y of age after controlling for covariates

(continued on next page)

Table 6 (continued)	
Stage of Life	**Mental Health Outcomes**

Adulthood	• A systematic review and meta-analysis of 13 cross-sectional and cohort studies concluded that healthy diet pattern was significantly associated with reduced odds of depression, but no statistically significant association was observed between unhealthy (Western) diet and depression (trend toward positive association)[39]
	• A meta-analysis of 22 studies investigated the association between a Mediterranean-style diet and brain diseases and determined that higher adherence to the Mediterranean-style diet was associated with reduced risk for depression and cognitive decline[40]
	Randomized controlled trial
	• Jacka and colleagues,[41] 2017, Supporting the Modification of lifestyle In Lowered Emotional States (SMILES) trial: included 67 adults diagnosed with depression; 31 in dietary support group and 25 in social support control group for 12 weeks
	  ○ The dietary support group received 7 60-min individual ModiMedDiet counseling sessions: diet rich in vegetables, fruit, and whole grains, with an emphasis on increased consumption of oily fish, extravirgin olive oil, legumes, and raw unsalted nuts, and moderate consumption of red meat and dairy
	  ○ The dietary support group showed significantly greater improvement in depressive symptoms between baseline and week 12 compared with the control group (32.3% vs 8%), number NNT based on remission score was 4.1 (95% CI of NNT, 2.3–27.8)
	  ○ All effects were independent of any changes in BMI, self-efficacy, smoking rates, and/or physical activity

Abbreviations: BMI, body mass index; CI, confidence interval; NNT, needed to treat.

Recommendations for Nutrition

The 1990 National Nutrition Monitoring and Related Research Act states that every 5 years the US Department of Agriculture (USDA) and Department of Health and Human Services must jointly publish dietary guidelines based on a preponderance of current scientific and medical knowledge. The 2015 to 2020 Dietary Guidelines for Americans marks the eighth edition and presents several changes from previous versions, including a change from MyPyramid to MyPlate (www.ChooseMyPlate.gov) as the guiding structure for nutritional decision making. The recommendations have increasingly acknowledged the importance of cultural needs as well as financial constraints. With emerging evidence, there are evolving updates for certain recommendations, including those for dietary cholesterol, fats, and calorie restriction:

- Loosening recommendations to limit dietary cholesterol (eg, eggs), but with caution because of frequent correlation between high cholesterol and high saturated fats in food.
- Reframing fats: not all fats are bad (eg, instead of avoiding all fats, move to reducing intake of saturated fatty acids by replacing them with monounsaturated fatty acids; eg, olive oil, nuts, avocados).
- Intermittent fasting and calorie restriction might have potential benefits in some adults; however, this is not recommended in children and adolescents given energy and growth requirements at this stage.

Table 7
Components of a nutritional assessment in the context of a mental health evaluation

Category	Sample Questions	Recommendations
What are they eating?	Are they: • Eating a variety of nutrient-dense foods? • Limiting processed foods that are high in added sugars, sodium, and saturated fat (eg, potato chips, fast food pizzas, white bread)? • Choosing water rather than juice and soda? • Showing any restrictions, aversions, or patterns of picky eating? • Taking vitamins and/or supplements?	• Shift focus from what not to eat to what to eat (eg, gradually replace candy/sweets with fruit, refined grain [eg, white bread] with whole grain, butter with olive oil, potato chips with kale chips or sweet potato fries) • Limit/avoid artificial sweeteners[53,54] (eg, choose water rather than diet soda) • If a child shows a pattern of picky eating, consider offering a choice between healthy food options (that the child might have helped pick in the store) in small, manageable portions in the context of an enjoyable environment in which all family members are eating the same meal (www.choosemyplate.gov) • Aim to obtain nutrients from food rather than supplements when possible (eg, drinking smoothies that include combinations of fruit, vegetables, and nuts, plus additional options of spices, oils, and seeds) • Include prebiotic (eg, bananas, garlic, onion) and probiotic foods (eg, fermented foods, yogurt) in the diet
Why are they eating?	Is the purpose of eating: • For nourishment/energy? • For enjoyment, craving? • To manage emotion, stress, boredom, or to provide comfort?	• Consider the role of mindful eating: making deliberate food choices and fully paying attention to the food[55] • Develop a list of healthy alternatives for comfort eating. In a study of college students there was no significant difference in resolution of negative feelings between groups that ate (1) comfort food, (2) liked-but-not-comforting food, or (3) plain granola bars[56]
With whom are they eating?	• What is the frequency and quality of family meals? • What is being modeled (eg, in the household)?	• Aim for at least 5 family meals per week (does not necessarily have to be dinner)[57] • Aim to make meals enjoyable experiences, choosing topics of conversation that foster engagement and interest • Encourage parents to increase awareness of their eating pattern and the impact it has not only on themselves but also on their children

(continued on next page)

Table 7 *(continued)*		
Category	**Sample Questions**	**Recommendations**
When do they eat?	• How often are they eating breakfast? • How about snacks? • What is the daily eating schedule?	• Problem-solve limitations to eating breakfast, because associations exist between having breakfast and improved student psychosocial and academic functioning[58] • Deliberately plan snack content and timing to manage energy needs of the child • Develop a list of acceptable healthy snacks and keep them readily available: Create a kids' snack drawer/cabinet that offers easily accessible healthy snacks; have fruits and vegetables precut and available for munching in a bowl on the counter/kitchen table
Where do they eat?	• Are they eating at the kitchen/dining room table? • How often are they eating in front of TV/screens? • How often are they eating at fast food restaurants?	• Maximize eating in spaces that promote mindful eating (eg, eat snacks at the kitchen table instead of in front of TV/computer/phone)

Although specific recommendations are likely to continue to change as knowledge and understanding of the interaction between food and the mind/body increase, a theme in current recommendations is to focus on a healthy eating pattern that is:

- High in fruits and vegetables (variety), whole grains, seafood, nuts, and legumes
- Moderate in low-fat dairy products
- Low in red and processed meat
- Very limited in processed foods, saturated fats and trans fats, added sugars, and sodium (unhealthy diet pattern)

As with changes in physical activity, improvement in dietary pattern can be challenging to accomplish quickly. Engaging the patient and family in motivational interviewing to help assess readiness to change (and first focusing on improving motivation to change if needed), identifying goals that are both appealing and manageable, and breaking goals down into small, incremental steps can increase the likelihood of success.[59] Opportunities for improved nutritional patterns through the who, what, when, why, and where of eating should be considered as part of psychiatric assessment and treatment planning and are included in **Table 7**.

SLEEP SCIENCE
Clinical Relevance and Current Research

Along with diet and exercise, sleep is an essential activity that plays a crucial role in emotional and physical development, health, and well-being. Quality sleep is associated with positive health and emotional outcomes in youth, including, but not limited to, improvements in attention, learning, academic performance, memory, cognition, behavior, and emotion regulation, as well as enhanced self-esteem, self-acceptance, levels of optimism, and overall quality of life.[60–62] In contrast, a wealth of evidence attests to the relationship between inadequate sleep and poorer health and emotional well-being in youth, including greater levels of self-criticism, internalizing symptoms, risk-taking behaviors, risk for suicidality and psychiatric illness, in addition to a host of negative effects on physical health and cognitive capabilities.[60,61,63–65]

Adequate sleep has been defined as the number of hours of daily sleep that an individual requires to function optimally and feel well rested.[66] Regrettably, most youth are not obtaining adequate sleep. Moreover, the likelihood that children will obtain adequate sleep decreases with age.[64] A survey of US students showed that nearly 60% of middle school students and nearly 75% of high school students endorsed short sleep duration on school nights (defined as <9 hours for children aged 6–12 years, or <8 hours for adolescents aged 13–18 years).[67] Similar results were found in a more recent study of high school students, with 71.9% reporting less than 8 hours of sleep per night.[65] In addition, this study found that the odds of engaging in risky behaviors (eg, risky driving, substance use, aggressive behaviors) increased as hours of sleep decreased.[65] Crucially, the strongest association was identified between sleep and mood and/or self-harm; youth who slept less than 6 hours per night were 3 times more likely to report suicidal behavior.[65]

Several factors contribute to poor sleep in youth, including electronic media exposure; caffeine consumption; early school start times; chronic medical conditions; neurologically based sleep disorders (eg, obstructive sleep apnea, restless legs syndrome); and pressures to achieve good grades, participate in extracurricular activities, and maintain an active social life.[64] Notably, youth from families of a lower socioeconomic status, as well as racial and ethnic minority youth, are at higher risk for insufficient sleep.[68,69] Sleep disruptions are frequently identified in children with psychiatric disorders, including attention-deficit/hyperactivity disorder, mood and disorders, and autism spectrum disorders.[63] The relationship between sleep and psychiatric illness is often bidirectional, whereby sleep disruptions are a symptom of a psychological disorder and the resulting poor sleep compounds and intensifies the condition.[63,70]

How It Works

Sleep architecture throughout most of childhood, adolescence, and adulthood consists of 2 stages: non–rapid eye movement sleep (NREM) and rapid eye movement sleep (REM), which are characterized by distinct electroencephalographic patterns and physiologic features. NREM sleep progresses through 3 stages of increasingly deep sleep and is considered necessary for rest and restoration. REM sleep follows stage 3 of NREM sleep, and is characterized by bouts of rapid eye movements, the suppression of muscle tone, and increases in brain activity, during which dreaming occurs. REM sleep is associated with dreaming, and is thought to play a role in the consolidation of memory and is crucial for the healthy development of the central nervous system. Children and adults enter sleep at stage 1 of NREM sleep and progress through NREM and REM cycles, which lengthen across development from 45 to 60 minutes in infancy to 90 to 110 minutes in childhood and adulthood, with brief periods of waking in between cycles. The amount of sleep necessary per 24-hour period peaks in neonates and decreases across childhood and adolescence.[71] **Table 8** outlines consensus guidelines from the American Academy of Sleep Medicine detailing the recommended amount of sleep in childhood and adolescence by age group.

Table 8
Recommended minimum and maximum hours of sleep recommended per age group within a 24-hour period

Age Group	Recommended Amount of Sleep per 24-h Period (h)
Infants 4–12 mo	12–16 (including naps)
Children 1–2 y	11–14 (including naps)
Children 3–5 y	10–13 (including naps)
Children 6–12 y	9–12
Teenagers 13–18 y	8–10

Adapted from Paruthi S, Brooks LJ, D'Ambrosio C, et al. Recommended amount of sleep for pediatric populations: a consensus statement of the American Academy of Sleep Medicine. J Clin Sleep Med 2016;12(6):785–6.

Clinical Assessment

Despite recommendations that sleep assessment be part of child well-visits, sleep is not regularly addressed in pediatric primary care.[72] It is therefore essential that mental health providers recognize the links between sleep and emotional well-being, and continuously assess and address sleep issues in the course of their work with youth. This assessment includes recognizing that both too little and too much sleep are associated with poorer outcomes.[61] Tools to assess pediatric sleep include clinical interviews, sleep diaries, and sleep questionnaires, such as the parent-report Children's Sleep Habits Questionnaire[73] or the adolescent-report School Sleep Habits Survey.[74] Clinicians should also assess environmental factors related to sleep quality and can be influential in assisting families to implement evidence-based behavioral recommendations to improve sleep. **Table 9** highlights potential areas of inquiry for parents or guardians to facilitate assessment of sleep hygiene and environmental factors. These questions can be modified to be asked directly of children as clinical context allows.

Recommendations for Sleep

Guidelines from the American Academy of Pediatrics detailed earlier can inform age-based recommendations for sleep duration, recognizing that the sleep needs of individual children may vary depending on the unique genetic, behavioral, medical, emotional, and environmental factors at play. In addition to recommendations about the duration of sleep, there are several environmental factors that should be considered, outlined in **Table 9**. In short, parents of children and adolescents should establish regular bedtimes and wake times to facilitate age-based recommendations for sleep duration. Implementing a consistent, predictable, and calming bedtime routine is particularly beneficial for children aged 12 years and younger.[60,75] Most research supports recommendations that sleep should occur:

- Independent of parental presence
- In a cool (16°–19°C [60°–67° F]), dark, comfortable, quiet room reserved primarily for sleeping[60]
- With minimal exposure to electronics, particularly in the evenings, and all electronic devices should be removed from children's rooms

In addition, sleep is optimized when children maintain a healthy diet, participate in regular physical activity, and have their emotional needs met during the day.[60] Some children require more targeted interventions to improve their sleep. Emerging evidence suggests that cognitive behavioral and mindfulness-based treatments may

Table 9
Sample questions to assess sleep hygiene in the context of a mental health evaluation and related recommendations

	Example Questions	Recommendations
Sleep Duration	• How long does the child sleep each night? • When is the child's bedtime during the week? On weekends? • How long does it take for the child to fall asleep at night? • Is the child napping? If yes, how frequently and for how long? • What is the child usually doing while waiting to fall asleep? (eg, listening to music, thinking about tomorrow, thinking about past events) • Is the child experiencing nighttime awakenings? If yes, how frequently and for how long?	• Adjust bedtimes and wake times to allow for age-appropriate sleep duration (see guidelines discussed earlier) • If it typically takes time for the child to fall asleep, set an earlier bedtime to permit the recommended amount of sleep (eg, a 13-y-old who wakes at 6 AM for school and takes 30 min to fall asleep should go to bed by 9:30 PM at the latest to ensure 8 h of nighttime sleep) • Keep bedtimes and wake times as consistent as possible on weeknights and weekends • Avoid daytime naps for children 6 y of age and older, unless the child is ill. Daytime naps for older children make it less likely that they will sleep at night • Encourage diaphragmatic breathing (belly breathing), progressive muscle relaxation, or other breathing-based relaxation strategies to facilitate sleep onset • For nighttime awakenings that last longer than 15 min, get out of bed and do a quiet activity (eg, reading, coloring) in dim light for 10 min, and then return to bed. This technique helps to reinforce that bed is associated only with sleep
Routines	• What is the child's daytime routine? (ie, meal times, school attendance, participation in extracurricular activities) • How consistent are the child's daytime and nighttime schedules? • Does the child have a wind-down or nighttime routine? (ie, shower, brush teeth, read a book, lights out) • Is the child's bed used for activities other than sleep, such as homework, watching TV, using the phone?	• Predictability during the day can help optimize nighttime sleep • Engaging in a consistent and calming bedtime routine can improve sleep; initiating the routine eventually cues the body that it is time for sleep via classic conditioning • Restrict caffeine intake beginning in the afternoon • Avoid exercising 3 h before bedtime • Avoid eating <2 h before bed, and limit liquid intake • Take a warm shower or bath before bed to relax. The change in body temperature from the warm water to the cool air also facilitates cooling of the body, which improves sleep • Listen to slow, relaxing music for 45 min before bedtime • The bed should be reserved only for sleep; avoid doing other activities on or in bed to reinforce the association between the bed and sleep

(continued on next page)

	Example Questions	Recommendations
Table 9 *(continued)*		
Sleep Environment	• Where does the child sleep in the home? • Does the child sleep alone? With siblings? With parents? • What is the child's sleep environment like? (eg, bright, noisy, comfortable, free of electronics)	• Whenever possible, sleep should occur independently (ie, in the child's own room) and in a dark room • Consider using white noise machines or fans to block sounds that may cause wakefulness • Sleep is optimized when the bedroom temperature is 16°–19°C [60°–67°F] (ie, the room should feel mildly chilly when you get out of bed) • Reduce exposure to blue light (ie, LED, florescent lights, screens) before bed; shift electronics to nighttime settings in the evening if they must be used before bed • Whenever possible, avoid exposure to screens entirely for 1–2 h before bedtime. Keep electronics away from the bed or bedside to avoid interruptions from notifications • Prevent viewing the clock by turning the clock face away or removing it entirely, because clockwatching can increase anxiety about not getting enough sleep

Abbreviation: LED, light-emitting diode.

be effective in addressing problems associated with poor sleep in at-risk youth.[76] When sleep problems do not respond to standard behavioral interventions, children should be referred for appropriate treatment.

Physical Activity, Nutrition, and Sleep Within a PERMA Framework

Because regular physical activity, balanced nutrition, and quality sleep are associated with improved well-being across the lifespan, it may be helpful for clinicians to adopt a framework that highlights the role of each lifestyle factor in optimizing well-being; one such framework is the PERMA model of mental well-being created by Martin Seligman, PhD.[15] This approach proposes that mental well-being is a multifactorial construct that includes the following elements[15]:

- P: positive emotions
- E: engagement
- R: relationships
- M: meaning
- A: accomplishments

The model further proposes a positive association between each of these elements and overall well-being. Clinicians may find it useful to consider PERMA elements during assessment and treatment to encourage children and adolescents to meet recommendations for physical activity, balanced nutrition, and sleep. **Table 10** offers example questions to address these PERMA factors in relation to each lifestyle factor. These questions can be modified to be asked of the parent as needed.

Table 10
Sample questions applying the PERMA wellness model to assess physical activity, nutrition, and sleep in the context of a mental health evaluation

PERMA Factor[15]	Sample Questions		
	Physical Activity	Nutrition	Sleep
Positive emotion	• What types of physical activity make you feel excited? Happy? Energized? • What positive emotions do you feel when you have finished working out? • How does exercising with other people, or playing a team sport, make you feel?	• Which meals make you feel content? Happy? Energized? Connected to others? • What are some of your favorite foods? • What positive emotions do you feel when you enjoy a nutritious meal? Is this any different from when you make less healthy choices?	• What is something you do before you go to bed that helps you to feel calm? • What positive emotions do you feel when you lie down in your bed to sleep at night? • How you feel when you wake up after a good night's sleep?
Engagement	• Which physical activities or sports best capture your interest? • What do you like about participating in team sports? How about individual sports? • Does competition help you push yourself, or impair your performance?	• Do you prepare meals yourself or with others? What are some of the benefits of both? • Where do you like to eat? Do you enjoy going to restaurants, or do you prefer eating meals at home? • What do you like to do while you are cooking? Do you listen to music, turn on the TV, talk to others? Or do you practice mindfulness while cooking?	• Do you look forward to sleeping? When you lie down, do you enjoy how your pillow and covers feel? Do you let go of your thoughts about the day to enjoy being in your bed? • What is a relaxing activity that you do before bed? Do you like to read a book, listen to calming music, or take a hot bath? • Is your bed the most comfortable place for you to sleep? Do you have several places where you feel so comfortable that it is easy for you to fall and stay asleep? • What is it like for you to do breathing exercises as you try and fall asleep?
Relationships	• Is there anyone with whom you like to exercise? • What team sports do you like to play? What is it like for you to be part of a sports team? • How does exercising with other people make you feel? Do you find that you push yourself more when you exercise with a partner?	• Who do you eat your meals with? Who do you enjoy eating with the most? • What sorts of things do you talk about when you eat meals with others? • How do you use meals to help build or support your relationships? Do you go out to dinner with friends, catch up with classmates over lunch in the cafeteria, or make meals with your family?	• How do you say goodnight to your family members before bed? • Do you feel safe and protected while you sleep? • Are there any books or songs that you share with others before bed?

(continued on next page)

Table 10
(continued)

PERMA Factor[15]	Sample Questions		
	Physical Activity	Nutrition	Sleep
Meaning	• What do you value about being physically active? Why is it important to you? • How do you feel about yourself when you are physically active on a regular basis? • What does winning or losing at a competitive physical activity mean to you? How does winning or losing affect you?	• Why does eating healthily matter to you? • Are there special meals that you and your family make during holidays or other special occasions? • What foods have meaning to you? Do any foods remind you of happy times, holidays, or special people?	• What is something that you have in your sleep environment/bedroom that is significant to you? A favorite stuffed animal? A picture of loved ones by your bed? • Do you value your sleep? Does it make you feel better? • Do you value and think or talk about your dreams?
Accomplishments	• Tell me about something that you accomplished that was physically challenging. How did you surprise yourself? • What is it like for you when you are part of a team that wins or performs well? • How do you think your schoolwork is affected by getting exercise? How about your social life?	• Do you feel a sense of pride when you make healthy food choices instead of unhealthy ones? • What is it like for you to prepare and eat a well-balanced meal?	• Do you notice any relationship between your sleep and your school performance (eg, paying attention in class)? • How does sleep affect how effective you are at getting things done the next day?

SUMMARY

The benefits conferred by physical activity, balanced nutrition, and quality sleep to youth physical well-being have generally been accepted. Emerging evidence continues to shed light on their benefits for youth mental health and wellness as well, including psychiatric disorders. These benefits seem to occur through multifactorial effects on neurobiological and psychosocial development. Integrating ongoing assessments and interventions related to these lifestyle domains within clinical practice promotes positive mental as well as physical health in youth, including enhancing treatment of psychiatric disorders and their impacts on functioning.

REFERENCES

1. Merikangas KR, He JP, Burstein M, et al. Lifetime prevalence of mental disorders in U.S. adolescents: results from the National Comorbidity Survey Replication— Adolescent Supplement (NCS-A). J Am Acad Child Adolesc Psychiatry 2010; 49(10):980–9.

2. Bailey AP, Hetrick SE, Rosenbaum S, et al. Treating depression with physical activity in adolescents and young adults: a systematic review and meta-analysis of randomised controlled trials. Psychol Med 2018;48(7):1068–83.

3. Halperin JM, Berwid OG, O'Neill S. Healthy body, healthy mind? The effectiveness of physical activity to treat ADHD in children. Child Adolesc Psychiatr Clin North Am 2014;23(4):899–936.

4. US Department of Health and Human Services. Physical activity guidelines for Americans. 2nd edition. Washington, DC: US Department of Health and Human Services; 2018.

5. Eime RM, Young JA, Harvey JT, et al. A systematic review of the psychological and social benefits of participation in sport for children and adolescents: informing development of a conceptual model of health through sport. Int J Behav Nutr Phys Act 2013;10:98.

6. Biddle SJ, Asare M. Physical activity and mental health in children and adolescents: a review of reviews. Br J Sports Med 2011;45(11):886–95.

7. Álvarez-Bueno C, Pesce C, Cavero-Redondo I, et al. The effect of physical activity interventions on children's cognition and metacognition: a systematic review and meta-analysis. J Am Acad Child Adolesc Psychiatry 2017;56(9):729–38.

8. Chaddock-Heyman L, Hillman CH, Cohen NJ, et al. The importance of physical activity and aerobic fitness for cognitive control and memory in children. Monogr Soc Res Child Dev 2014;79(4):25–50.

9. Chaddock L, Erickson KI, Prakash RS, et al. A neuroimaging investigation of the association between aerobic fitness, hippocampal volume, and memory performance in preadolescent children. Brain Res 2010;1358:172–83.

10. Schuch FB, Vancampfort D, Firth J, et al. Physical activity and incident depression: a meta-analysis of prospective cohort studies. Am J Psychiatry 2018; 175(7):631–48.

11. Carter T, Morres ID, Meade O, et al. The effect of exercise on depressive symptoms in adolescents: a systematic review and meta-analysis. J Am Acad Child Adolesc Psychiatry 2016;55(7):580–90.

12. Klein JB, Jacobs RH, Reinecke MA. Cognitive-behavioral therapy for adolescent depression: a meta-analytic investigation of changes in effect-size estimates. J Am Acad Child Adolesc Psychiatry 2007;46(11):1403–13.

13. Whittington CJ, Kendall T, Fonagy P, et al. Selective serotonin reuptake inhibitors in childhood depression: systematic review of published versus unpublished data. Lancet 2004;363(9418):1341–5.

14. Sibold J, Edwards E, Murray-Close D, et al. Physical activity, sadness, and suicidality in bullied US adolescents. J Am Acad Child Adolesc Psychiatry 2015; 54(10):808–15.

15. Seligman MEP. Authentic happiness: using the new positive psychology to realize your potential for lasting fulfillment. New York: Free Press; 2002.

16. Taliaferro LA, Rienzo BA, Pigg RM Jr, et al. Associations between physical activity and reduced rates of hopelessness, depression, and suicidal behavior among college students. J Am Coll Health 2009;57(4):427–36.

17. Stavrakakis N, de Jonge P, Ormel J, et al. Bidirectional prospective associations between physical activity and depressive symptoms. The TRAILS Study. J Adolesc Health 2012;50(5):503–8.

18. Hoza B, Martin CP, Pirog A, et al. Using physical activity to manage ADHD symptoms: the state of the evidence. Curr Psychiatry Rep 2016;18(12):113.

19. Rommel AS, Lichtenstein P, Rydell M, et al. Is physical activity causally associated with symptoms of attention-deficit/hyperactivity disorder? J Am Acad Child Adolesc Psychiatry 2015;54(7):565–70.

20. Terry-McElrath YM, O'Malley PM, Johnston LD. Exercise and substance use among American youth, 1991-2009. Am J Prev Med 2011;40(5):530–40.

21. Koivukangas J, Tammelin T, Kaakinen M, et al. Physical activity and fitness in adolescents at risk for psychosis within the Northern Finland 1986 Birth Cohort. Schizophr Res 2010;116(2–3):152–8.

22. Cote AT, Devlin AM, Panagiotopoulos C. Initial screening of children treated with second-generation antipsychotics points to an association between physical activity and insulin resistance. Pediatr Exerc Sci 2014;26(4):455–62.

23. Vopat BG, Klinge SA, McClure PK, et al. The effects of fitness on the aging process. J Am Acad Orthop Surg 2014;22(9):576–85.

24. Lubans D, Richards J, Hillman C, et al. Physical activity for cognitive and mental health in youth: a systematic review of mechanisms. Pediatrics 2016;138(3) [pii: e20161642].

25. GBD 2015 Obesity Collaborators, Afshin A, Forouzanfar MH, Reitsma MB, et al. Health effects of overweight and obesity in 195 countries over 25 years. N Engl J Med 2017;377(1):13–27.

26. Sartori SB, Whittle N, Hetzenauer A, et al. Magnesium deficiency induces anxiety and HPA axis dysregulation: modulation by therapeutic drug treatment. Neuropharmacology 2012;62(1):304–12.

27. Torabi M, Kesmati M, Harooni HE, et al. Effects of nano and conventional zinc oxide on anxiety-like behavior in male rats. Indian J Pharmacol 2013;45(5):508–12.

28. Kiecolt-Glaser JK, Belury MA, Andridge R, et al. Omega-3 supplementation lowers inflammation and anxiety in medical students: a randomized controlled trial. Brain Behav Immun 2011;25(8):1725–34.

29. Jacka FN, Cherbuin N, Kaarin J, et al. Western diet is associated with a smaller hippocampus: a longitudinal investigation. BMC Med 2015;13:215.

30. Pina-Camacho L, Jensen SK, Gaysina D, et al. Maternal depression symptoms, unhealthy diet and child emotional-behavioural dysregulation. Psychol Med 2015;45(9):1851–60.

31. Steenweg-de Graaff J, Tiemeier H, Steegers-Theunissen RP, et al. Maternal dietary patterns during pregnancy and child internalising and externalising problems. The Generation R Study. Clin Nutr 2014;33(1):115–21.

32. Jacka FN, Ystrom E, Brantsaeter AL, et al. Maternal and early postnatal nutrition and mental health of offspring by age 5 years: a prospective cohort study. J Am Acad Child Adolesc Psychiatry 2013;52(10):1038–47.
33. Khalid S, Williams CM, Reynolds SA. Is there an association between diet and depression in children and adolescents? A systematic review. Br J Nutr 2017; 116(12):2097–108.
34. Jacka FN, Kremer PJ, Berk M, et al. A prospective study of diet quality and mental health in adolescents. PLoS One 2011;6(9):e24805.
35. McMartin SE, Kuhle S, Colman I, et al. Diet quality and mental health in subsequent years among Canadian youth. Public Health Nutr 2012;15(12):2253–8.
36. Jacka FN, Rothon C, Taylor S, et al. Diet quality and mental health problems in adolescents from East London: a prospective study. Soc Psychiatry Psychiatr Epidemiol 2013;48:1297–306.
37. Trapp GS, Allen KL, Black LJ, et al. A prospective investigation of dietary patterns and internalizing and externalizing mental health problems in adolescents. Food Sci Nutr 2016;4(6):888–96.
38. Winpenny EM, van Harmelen AL, White M, et al. Diet quality and depressive symptoms in adolescence: no cross-sectional or prospective associations following adjustment for covariates. Public Health Nutr 2018;21(13):2376–84.
39. Lai JS, Hiles S, Bisquera A, et al. A systematic review and meta-analysis of dietary patterns and depression in community-dwelling adults. Am J Clin Nutr 2014; 99(1):181–97.
40. Psaltopoulou T, Sergentanis TN, Panagiotakos DB, et al. Mediterranean diet, stroke, cognitive impairment, and depression: a meta-analysis. Ann Neurol 2013;74:580–91.
41. Jacka FN, O'Neil A, Opie R, et al. A randomized controlled trial of dietary improvement for adults with major depression (the 'SMILES' trial). BMC Med 2017;15:23.
42. Shivappa N, Hebert JR, Tehrani AN, et al. A pro-inflammatory diet is associated with an increased odds of depression symptoms among Iranian female adolescents: a cross-sectional study. Front Psychiatry 2018;9:400.
43. Moylan S, Berk M, Dean OM, et al. Oxidative & nitrosative stress in depression: Why so much stress? Neurosci Biobehav Rev 2014;45C:46–62.
44. Murphy T, Dias GP, Thuret S. Effects of diet on brain plasticity in animal and human studies: mind the gap. Neural Plast 2014;2014:563160.
45. Akbaraly T, Sexton C, Zsoldos E, et al. Association of long-term diet quality with hippocampal volume: longitudinal cohort study. Am J Med 2018;131(11): 1372–81.e4.
46. Cryan JF, Dinan TG. Mind-altering microorganisms: the impact of the gut microbiota on brain and behaviour. Nat Rev Neurosci 2012;13(10):701–12.
47. Valdes AM, Walter J, Segal E, et al. Role of the gut microbiota in nutrition and health. BMJ 2018;361:k2179.
48. Cerdo T, Ruiz A, Suarez A, et al. Probiotic, prebiotic, and brain development. Nutrients 2017;9(11):1247.
49. Dash S, Clarke G, Berk M, et al. The gut microbiome and diet in psychiatry: focus on depression. Curr Opin Psychiatry 2015;28(1):1–6.
50. David LA, Maurice CF, Carmody RN, et al. Diet rapidly and reproducibly alters the human gut microbiome. Nature 2014;505:559–63.
51. De Filippo C, Cavalieri D, Di Paola M, et al. Impact of diet in shaping gut microbiota revealed by a comparative study in children from Europe and rural Africa. Proc Natl Acad Sci U S A 2010;107:14691–6.

52. Scaglioni S, Arrizza C, Vecchi F, et al. Determinants of children's eating behavior. Am J Clin Nutr 2011;94(6 Suppl):2006S–11S.

53. Pearlman M, Obert J, Casey L. The association between artificial sweeteners and obesity. Curr Gastroenterol Rep 2017;19(12):64.

54. Swithers SE. Artificial sweeteners are not the answer to childhood obesity. Appetite 2015;93:85–90.

55. Dalen J, Smith BW, Shelley BM, et al. Pilot study: Mindful Eating and Living (MEAL): weight, eating behavior, and psychological outcomes associated with a mindfulness-based intervention for people with obesity. Complement Ther Med 2010;18(6):260–4.

56. Wagner H, Ahlstrom B, Redden JP, et al. The myth of comfort food. Health Psychol 2014;33(12):1552–7.

57. Haghighatdoost F, Kelishadi R, Qorbani M, et al. Dinner frequency is inversely related to mental disorders and obesity in adolescents: the CASPIAN-III study. Arch Iran Med 2017;20(4):218–23.

58. Murphy JM, Pagano ME, Nachmani J, et al. The relationship of school breakfast to psychosocial and academic functioning: cross-sectional and longitudinal observations in an inner-city school sample. Arch Pediatr Adolesc Med 1998; 152(9):899–907.

59. Horwath CC. Applying the transtheoretical model to eating behavior change: challenges and opportunities. Nutr Res Rev 1999;12:281–317.

60. Allen SL, Howlett MD, Coulombe JA, et al. ABCs of SLEEPING: a review of the evidence behind pediatric sleep practice recommendations. Sleep Med Rev 2016;29:1–14.

61. Paruthi S, Brooks LJ, D'Ambrosio CD, et al. Recommended amount of sleep for pediatric populations: a consensus statement of the American Academy of Sleep Medicine. J Clin Sleep Med 2016;12(6):785–6.

62. Sampasa-Kanyinga H, Standage M, Tremblay MS, et al. Associations between meeting combinations of 24-h movement guidelines and health-related quality of life in children from 12 countries. Public Health 2017;153:16–24.

63. Alfano CA, Gamble AL. The role of sleep in childhood psychiatric disorders. Child Youth Care Forum 2009;38(6):327–40.

64. Owens JA, Adolescent Sleep Working Group, Committee of Adolescence. Insufficient sleep in adolescents and young adults: an update on causes and consequences. Pediatrics 2014;134(3):e921–32.

65. Weaver MD, Barger LK, Malone SK, et al. Dose-dependent association between sleep duration and unsafe behaviors among US high school students. JAMA Pediatr 2018;172(12):1187–9.

66. Williams JA, Zimmerman FJ, Bell JF. Norms and trends of sleep time among US children and adolescents. JAMA Pediatr 2013;167(1):55–60.

67. Wheaton AG, Jones SE, Cooper AC, et al. Short sleep duration among middle school and high school students – United States, 2015. MMWR Morb Mortal Wkly Rep 2018;67(3):85–9.

68. Marco CA, Wolfson AR, Sparling M, et al. Family socioeconomic status and sleep patterns of young adolescents. Behav Sleep Med 2011;10(1):70–80.

69. Spilsbury JC, Storfer-Isser A, Drotar D, et al. Sleep behavior in an urban US sample of school-aged children. Arch Pediatr Adolesc Med 2004;158(10):988–94.

70. Lofthouse N, Gilchrist R, Splaingard M. Mood-related sleep problems in children and adolescents. Child Adolesc Psychiatr Clin North Am 2009;18(4):893–916.

71. Bathory E, Tomopoulous S. Sleep regulation, physiology and development, sleep durations and patterns, and sleep hygiene in infants, toddlers, and preschool-age children. Curr Probl Pediatr Adolesc Health Care 2017;47:29–42.
72. Honaker SM, Meltzer LJ. Sleep in pediatric primary care: a review of the literature. Sleep Med Rev 2016;25:31–9.
73. Owens JA, Spirito A, McGuinn M. The Children's Sleep Habits Questionnaire (CSHQ): psychometric properties of a survey instrument for school-aged children. Sleep 2000;23:1–9.
74. Wolfson AR, Carskadon MA. Sleep schedules and daytime functioning in adolescents. Child Dev 1998;69:875–87.
75. Mindell JA, Williamson AA. Benefits of a bedtime routine in young children: sleep, development, and beyond. Sleep Med Rev 2018;40:93–108.
76. Blake MJ, Snoep L, Raniti M, et al. A cognitive-behavioral and mindfulness-based group sleep intervention improves behavior problems in at-risk adolescents by improving perceived sleep quality. Behav Res Ther 2017;99:147–56.

Make a Joyful Noise
Integrating Music into Child Psychiatry Evaluation and Treatment

Jeff Q. Bostic, MD, EdD[a],*, Christopher R. Thomas, MD[b],
Eugene V. Beresin, MD[c],[1], Anthony L. Rostain, MD, MA[d],
David L. Kaye, MD[e]

KEYWORDS

- Mental health • Well-being • Music • Child and adolescent

KEY POINTS

- Music is the most common nonschool activity of youth, occupying approximately 4 hours per day. Music triggers specific brain pathways associated with pleasure, reward, arousal, and decreases activity in harm/avoidance/risk appraisal pathways.
- Playing music improves general cognitive ability, reading ability, visuospatial skills, self-esteem, school engagement, and decreases behavioral difficulties and aggression.
- Musical preferences can quickly be identified by their impacts on arousal (vs calming) and attractive (vs avoiding). Music is helpful for decreasing anxiety, specifically when undergoing medical procedures.
- In school/work environments, music that is soft, slow, instrumental, and low intensity can be helpful during student practice/homework activities.
- Music practice is most effective when all body parts are used to play the section, difficult sections are played slowly at first so they can be played correctly with attention to how they sound musically, and then different parts are connected so that the piece flows together.

Disclosure Statement: None.
The authors acknowledge that they are members of the band Pink Freud.
[a] Department of Psychiatry, MedStar Georgetown University Hospital, 2115 Wisconsin Avenue, Northwest, Suite 200, Washington, DC 20007, USA; [b] Department of Psychiatry and Behavioral Sciences, University of Texas Medical Branch-Galveston, 301 University Boulevard, Galveston, TX 77555-0193, USA; [c] Department of Psychiatry, Massachusetts General Hospital, Harvard University, 55 Fruit St., Boston, MA 02114, USA; [d] Department of Psychiatry, Perelman School of Medicine, University of Pennsylvania, 3535 Market Street, Room 2007, Philadelphia, PA 19104, USA; [e] Department of Psychiatry, University at Buffalo Jacobs School of Medicine, 462 Grider St, Buffalo NY 14215, USA
[1] 80 School Street; Acton, MA 01720.
* Corresponding author.
E-mail address: Jeffrey.q.bostic@gunet.georgetown.edu

Child Adolesc Psychiatric Clin N Am 28 (2019) 195–207
https://doi.org/10.1016/j.chc.2018.11.003
1056-4993/19/© 2018 Elsevier Inc. All rights reserved.

Abbreviations	
NA	Nucleus accumbens
PERMA	Positive Emotions, Engagement, Relationships, Meaning, Accomplishment

Music is the medicine of the mind

—John Logan

Music amplifies emotions, intensifying the human experience. Music affords an accessible means for young people to recognize and express emotions, connects diverse people (through sharing preferred music, becoming exhilarated by concerts, etc), and embeds memories (as music becomes associated with one's life events). Music can provide alternative opportunities for youth to express their feelings. As Hans Christian Anderson remarked, "Where words fail, music speaks."

Clinically, child psychiatrists usually seek various approaches for youth to establish adaptive patterns that can yield positive emotions, more effective engagement in activities, better connections with others, meaningful experiences and expression, and significant life accomplishments. Child psychiatrists can help patients to identify which music best soothes their sometimes-ravaged souls. And beyond listening, brain science findings now reveal what type of "practice" is most effective to learn how to sing or play an instrument.

MUSIC AND THE DEVELOPING BRAIN
Listening to Music

Hearing and enjoying music seems to be universal. Cambodians unfamiliar with Western rock music had the same emotional reactions to rock music as Westerners.[1] Humans seem to be wired to understand music; like reading, humans across cultures naturally make sense of music, follow chord changes, and remember melodies.[2] Humans similarly seem to be wired to enjoy music, naturally releasing dopamine at peak (climax) moments in music.[3]

The brain begins to enjoy music within the first year of life as motor neurons become activated during passive listening.[4] By age 20 to 30 years, brain pathways are associated with musical responses[5]:

1. *Euphoria/pleasant emotion pathways* in the nucleus accumbens (NA), ventral tegmental area, anterior cingulate, and insula;
2. *Reward pathways* (similarly to responses to food/sex/drugs) through dopamine activity in the NA, ventral tegmental area, and opioid receptors in periaqueductal gray and pedunculopontine nucleus;
3. *Arousal pathways* in the insula, thalamus, anterior cingulate; and
4. *Evaluation of reward/punishment pathways* in the orbitofrontal regions.

At the same time, music decreases activity in the harm/avoidance/risk appraisal pathways through decreased cholinergic activity in the amygdala, hippocampus, and ventral medial prefrontal cortex. Stimulating music increases activity in the NA, ventral tegmental area, orbital frontal cortex, and insula, and decreases activity in the amygdala (**Fig. 1**).

Playing Music and Brain Functioning

Playing music seems to be more beneficial than listening, just as playing sports yields more benefits than watching them.[6] Multiple cognitive skills benefit from playing an

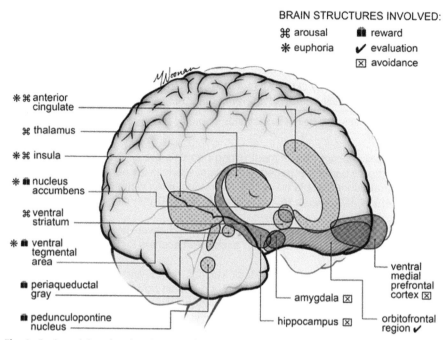

BRAIN STRUCTURES INVOLVED:

⌘ arousal   🎁 reward
✳ euphoria   ✔ evaluation
                 ☒ avoidance

✳⌘ anterior
     cingulate

⌘ thalamus

✳⌘ insula

✳🎁 nucleus
     accumbens

⌘ ventral
     striatum

✳🎁 ventral
     tegmental
     area   ventral
                                             medial
🎁 periaqueductal   prefrontal
     gray   amygdala ☒   cortex ☒

🎁 pedunculopontine   orbitofrontal
     nucleus   hippocampus ☒   region ✔

Fig. 1. Brain activity when hearing stimulating music. (*Courtesy of* M. Noonan, MSMI, CMI, Arlington, VA.)

instrument. Metaanalytic studies show improved visual-spatial skills in those who played an instrument.[7] At 24 weeks of musical instrument practice, general reading ability improved in third graders,[8] and at 36 weeks of practice, general cognitive abilities were improved in 6-year-olds.[9] Kraus and colleagues[6] found that 7- to 10-year-old students playing an instrument for 28 to 39 h/y (vs those attending a music appreciation class) developed greater reading proficiency. Practicing an instrument also increases cortical thickness, particularly in the attention, premotor, motor regions.[10]

Across cultures, social-emotional skills and capacities are enhanced by playing musical instruments. Researchers have reported improved self-esteem,[11] and school engagement[12] among students who play musical instruments. Music training improves self-control, reduces behavioral difficulties,[13] and improves self-esteem.[14] Performing yielded greater benefits than rehearsals.[15]

Lyrics

Some people listen to music and essentially ignore lyrics, whereas for others the converse is true. Melodies have more impact than lyrics on one's experience of both positive and negative emotions. However, lyrics have been shown to detract from happy/positive emotion-inducing melodies, but enhance sad/negative emotion-inducing melodies.[16] Several high-profile lawsuits contended that certain types of music or lyrics increased suicidality. The evidence has found that suicidality is more likely related to other personality traits or psychiatric symptoms of those who suicide than their musical preferences.[17]

Music Anhedonia

Approximately 3% to 5% of people have a specific music anhedonia, and do not enjoy music, despite being able to derive pleasure from other things such as food, drink, and other activities. Decreased activity in the NA and decreased connectivity between the ventral striatum and right auditory cortex (supratemporal gyrus) suggests that their auditory and reward centers do not interact.[18]

INTEGRATING MUSIC INTO CLINICAL EVALUATION AND TREATMENT
Inquiring about Musical Interests/Preferences in Young People

Several lines of evidence favor the inclusion of music in clinical evaluations and treatment with youth:

1. Music is a significant part of most young people's lives.[19] Youth spend approximately 4 hours per day engaged with music. Music is the number one nonschool activity that young people do each day, not including watching videos (eg, YouTube), which now seems to occupy more than 60 min/d for young people as well.
2. Young people listen to music in multiple public and private settings compared with adults. Music plays a greater role in social relationships for youth compared with adults.[19]
3. Adolescents use music as part of their identity, values, and beliefs.[20] The musical attachments one forms during adolescence remain powerful throughout life, in a shared musical lexicon and cultural experience.
4. Music is well-associated with altering mood states, quickly. Indeed, this has been recognized and is now commonly used among athletes to titrate their emotions during games.[21]
5. Music remains a preferred tactic for people of all ages to manage stress.[22]

Music Items for the Mental Health Evaluation

Child clinicians may most easily embed a few broad questions into their clinical interview to discern (1) the importance of music, as well as (2) opportunities to use music to enhance well-being, for each patient.

Evaluation of musical preferences
Evaluation of 3 components of musical preferences may aid in planning subsequent treatment.

1. Current musical preferences: Most young people describe preferred songs, musicals, groups, or styles of music; some will describe lyrics that resonate with them or provide special meaning.
2. Reactions to unfamiliar music: Youth will often listen to unfamiliar music and describe their reactions to it, both allowing opportunities for extension of current preferences, and for connection with treaters around common music, themes, or artist interests.
3. Participation in music: Gallup[23] polls indicate that more than one-half of all households have someone who plays music and that 82% began playing by the age of 14. European data indicate that about 77% of children will play an instrument during childhood, peaking at ages 8 to 10 and then decreasing to approximately 60% by ages 16 to 17.[24]

Although more formal assessments of emotional reactions to music are available (eg, the Geneva Emotional Music Scale[25,26]), a simple approach follows classifying music on 2 axes by arousal versus calming and attractive versus avoidance[27] (**Fig. 2**).

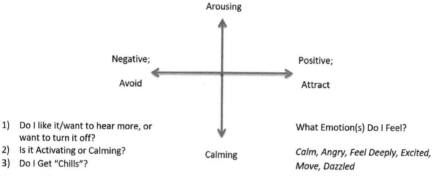

1) Do I like it/want to hear more, or want to turn it off?
2) Is it Activating or Calming?
3) Do I Get "Chills"?

What Emotion(s) Do I Feel?

Calm, Angry, Feel Deeply, Excited, Move, Dazzled

Fig. 2. Evaluating pieces of music.

Evaluation of reactions to music

For patients who show interest in music and affix meaning to music, **Table 1** provides questions for clinicians to consider addressing during the interview (or as part of screening, patient/parents may complete prior to an interview). Items are categorized by the PERMA categories (*Positive Emotions, Engagement, Relationships, Meaning, Accomplishment*) described by Seligman,[28] and can be individualized to the needs and interests of the patients. Not all of these questions are feasible, so various items may be used or adjusted to clarify musical engagement and opportunities within treatment. For example, if a patient is struggling with negative emotions, then the Positive Emotions questions may be more useful, whereas another patient may struggle with relationships and benefit from Relationship questions.

INCORPORATING MUSIC INTO CLINICAL TREATMENT

The PERMA categories described in Table 1 suggest a framework for clinical applications.

Positive Emotions and Music

Music is the divine way to tell beautiful, poetic things to the heart.

—*Pablo Casals*

Music evokes all types of emotions, from positive to neutral (eg, background music) to negative emotions. A patient's interest in sad music can illuminate that others (who wrote/played it) have experienced this emotion as well, contributing to connections. Helping patients to recognize what about the music (tempo, melody, lyrics, etc) amplifies their experience can be helpful. Clarifying which music evokes positive emotions is also important, because this information can help patients to engage or transition around difficult circumstances. Music varies for individuals, as some may describe feeling "fired up" when listening to music that others describe as "scary" or "intense." The goals for the clinician regarding music and positive emotions are:

- To help patients identify music which enhances or brings about positive emotions; and
- To help patients identify particular musical pieces to augment or alter a current mood state (eg, create their playlist to shift up for activities or down to transition into the evening and sleep).

Table 1 Integrating music into the well-being interview	
Significance	1. What *place* does music have in your life? 2. How do you *use* music in your life? 3. How often do you "*go to*" music at times during your day? 4. Is music a *regular* part of your day? (times when you listen or play music)
Positive emotions	What songs make you: 1. *Calm?* (slow you down) 2. *Angry?* (make you want to lash out) 3. *Feel deeply?* (sadness, joy, etc) 4. *Excited?* (motivate you) 5. *Move?* (dance, get activated) 6. *Dazzled?* (awe/amaze you)
Engagement	1. Do you listen mostly to the *music or* more to the *lyrics*? 2. How do *lyrics affect* you? 3. Do you *sing, hum, or whistle* tunes? 4. Do you *play* (or plan to play) an instrument or *sing*? 5. If you could be in a *band*, which one would it be? 6. How do you *learn about new music* that might appeal to you?
Flow	1. Do you ever "*lose yourself*" in music (lose time, forget about all else)? 2. What (all) *leads to losing yourself* in that moment (listening to particular songs, singing along, playing, practicing, playing with others)?
Relationships	Do you: 1. *Listen* to music *with others*? 2. *Share* music with others? 3. Go to *concerts with others*? 4. *Play music with others*? Has music: 1. Brought you *closer to others*? 2. *Connected you to anyone* you want to know more about/be like in some way? 3. *Changed your opinion* about someone (based on their musical preferences)? 4. *Reminded* you of others or past experiences?
Meaning	Do you: 1. *Spend much time* with music in your life? 2. *Learn new things* from music? 3. See *influences* in your life by songs or musicians? 4. Feel *inspired* to do/try new or different things? 5. *Remember* songs ("want to use that for my wedding")?
Accomplishment	Do you: 1. *Associate music* with any of your achievements? 2. Identify *successes* you have had in music performance? 3. Think music has *helped you deal with* anything? 4. Feel like music/musicians have encouraged you to *stretch*?

Music and Mood Regulation

Clinically, the effort is to encourage patients to identify music that is both desirable to listen to and improves distressing moods. Creating a playlist where the patient can select appropriate music may help to regulate mood and decrease the stress hormone cortisol.[29] Music improves distress and anxiety for those, including pediatric patients, awaiting[30,31] or undergoing medical procedures, even rivaling medication interventions.[32,33]

Music can also make one feel more hopeful after failure experiences.[34] Music has now been "created" to decrease anxiety; for example, Mindlab International has reported notable decreases in anxiety in adults listening to soft, slow instrumental music with minimal lyrics, such as "Weightless" by Marconi Union, which was created to slow the listener's heart rate, lower blood pressure, and diminish cortisol release.

Listening to Sad Music

Red, white, black, brown, yellow, rich, poor, we all have the blues.

—BB King

Parents often worry that listening to negative or sad music will only worsen their child's mood. Listening to sad music itself is often described as evoking multiple emotions, including those that intensify pleasure.[35] Sad music releases endorphins, which induce prolactin release, which is associated with gratification and relaxation.[36] Sad music also suggests that one is not alone, because indeed someone else is experiencing and conveying their (perhaps similar) sadness through music, and similar emotions between us seems to be comforting.[37]

Engagement

Life seems to go on without effort when I am filled with music.

—George Eliot

Musical engagement refers to (1) how much music is part of one's life, and (2) the impact music has, in that moment, in one's life. First, how much one notices or listens to music, or whether they regularly sing or play and instrument, may clarify receptivity to integration of these PERMA components in treatment. Second, some young patients may "dutifully" practice an instrument, whereas others readily listen, sing, or play music and "lose themselves" (eg, lose track of time) when they engage with the music.

Music in the Classroom (or While Doing Homework)

Music is distracting during instruction,[38] but can be helpful while students are doing homework, writing, drawing, or practicing spelling words[39] or to decrease ambient noise (eg, students talking, hallway noise, etc). Classical and soft jazz instrumental music seem to be most appropriate, and may be particularly helpful for students reactive to sudden or distracting noise (eg, for students with attention deficit hyperactivity disorder, past trauma, etc), and "no noise" (eg, headphones) may also be helpful for these students. Background music that is instrumental, slow tempo, soft volume, and low intensity seems to be most helpful in the classroom.[40] Music in the classroom is more distracting when it is loud,[41] fast,[42] highly liked or disliked, or more intense.[43] Music containing lyrics is unhelpful and distracting,[44] unless the lyrics themselves are educationally relevant, such as the "alphabet song" (where singing and rhyming the letters helps to enhance recall). Educational songs, more popular among young students, are available at sites such as https://www.wondershare.com/songsdownload/top-50-educational-songs-free-download.html.

Relationships

Music is the great reunite. . . . Something that people who differ on everything and anything else can have in common.

—Sarah Dressen

People of all ages report increased interpersonal trust and bonding while listening to music.[45,46] Music shared among young adolescents made experiences more positive, except when listening to music with family members.[47] Music sharing among adolescents enhances social interactions, so helping adolescent patients to identify which music to share with particular peers may help adolescents to connect with peers. Music increases receptivity to relationships. Singing (amateurs or professionals) raises oxytocin levels immediately after a 30-minute singing experience,[48] and women listening to romantic music are much more likely (52% vs 28%) to agree to go out on a date.[49]

Meaning
Music is the greatest communication in the world. Even if people don't understand the language you're singing in, they still know good music when they hear it.

—Lou Rawls

Music "sticks" with us and may alter how we see the world around us. Most listeners derive both similar meanings and have similar emotional reactions, particularly in musical reactions to feeling happiness, sadness, anger, and tenderness.[50] Reimer[51] has described 5 characteristics contributing to the power of music.

1. Music is both a "means" of expression and an "end," with a product that can be replayed to remind us of experiences or to evoke emotions. Clinically, this may allow patients to both use music, songs, and lyrics to express that which most matters to them, and to identify works which rekindle or alter past experiences. Exploring what preferred music represents or recalls for patients allows another vehicle to understanding.
2. Music encompasses mind, body, and feeling. Like the cognitive triad (thought, feeling, action), music may arouse thought, evoke feelings, or influence actions (eg, dance, "drum," or play). Clinically, exploring what music entices a patient to feel or do, provides an opportunity to help the patient identify beneficial musical "triggers" for positive thoughts, feelings, and actions.
3. Music is simultaneously universal, cultural, and individual. Clinically, music may retain personal meaning or represent a cultural awareness or movement meaningful to a particular time ("yes, that was our music that reflected our time").
4. Music is both a "process" and a "product." The process of making music is as meaningful as listening to the finished project (changes in the arrangements, lyrics, tempos, etc, may perpetuate this process). Clinically, replaying or identifying similar music may increase sensation and meaning. Finding preferred music played by alternative groups, or alternative versions (eg, live, same song at different tempos, etc), may induce different reactions.
5. Music is pleasurable and profound. Some reactions can only be evoked by music. Clinically, reviewing with patients what "new" experiences occur when hearing new (desirable) music, and how their experiences change with different music may provide different routes to address previously distressing emotions.

Accomplishment
The most joy in my life has come to me from my violin.

—Albert Einstein

Accomplishment may be as direct as a patient finding music that enhances mood, or developing a playlist that enhances exercise, meal times, or daily routine tasks. A more difficult, but rewarding, accomplishment involves creating music, made easier now with software where one can create without actually playing instruments. Being able to play an instrument yields another form of accomplishment, as one masters and commands a tool (be it voice or instrument).

Creating music with others enhances connection, engagement, positive emotion, and sense of well-being. Moreover, one can make a difference when contributing to the sound of a band. Improvisation may further express individuality and stimulate other players. This process can help in the developmental task of adolescence of becoming one's own person and still feeling a part of a group.

Practical Applications

In this section, tactics are described for enhancing benefits from music practice, and which extrapolate to other situations (eg, shooting a basketball, etc).

Effective musical practice

Too often, when one starts playing an instrument, the emphasis is on practicing "30 minutes a day." Duke and colleagues[52] studied young adult pianists to discern what matters during practice (summarized in **Table 2**).

To gain the most from music practice:

- Use both hands (feet) needed to play the section,
- Think about the piece musically (how it will sound best),
- Work out difficult sections slowly and gradually speed them up, and then
- Connect the parts of the piece so that all the parts flow together.

What is not helpful is to practice for some fixed length of time, play through the entire piece without stopping to work out difficult parts or errors, or to play the piece some certain number of times.

It takes longer for some to develop technical proficiency, but it is not how many notes or how fast one can play the piece—it is how notes played sound to others. Recording oneself and listening to how a part sounds, and also to how it blends with others (parts and other players), can be very helpful. Performing (in front of others) and gauging and inquiring how it sounded is also helpful.

Table 2
Factors influencing effective musical practice

What Helps	What Hinders
Higher percentage of times played correctly	Number of times played incorrectly
Using both hands/all appendages	Playing through difficult sections and making mistakes
Using musical inflection from beginning	Playing the notes on the page even if it sounds badly
Thinking musically (humming, singing it as it should sound, etc)	Focusing on one's part and not listening to others to ebb and flow (tempo, volume) with the other musicians
Playing difficult sections slowly and correctly and then increasing tempo	Playing through difficult sections quickly to get to the easier sections
Focusing on difficult parts or mistakes and working, slowly on those	Focusing on the easier parts and practicing as much or more on those than difficult parts
Correcting problem parts until smooth	"Getting it right once" and presuming every time thereafter one will play it correctly as well

Reading music

You can't teach me. Everyone has tried, starting with my mother. I have some kind of block. I'm not alone. There are a lot of guys who have a name like mine who can't read music.

—Dave Brubeck

Considerable controversy surrounds the benefits of reading music ("learning from sheet music") versus listening ("learning by ear"). SI Hayakawa commented that "the map is not the land; the word is not the thing," and the notes on the page are not the sounds. Thinking one played the part "well" because one followed the "map" (sheet music) does not make it sound good.

A number of great musicians resisted learning to read music, fearing it would alter how they play music. Eric Clapton, Michael Jackson, Paul McCartney (and the other Beatles), Jimi Hendrix, Eddie Van Halen, Ry Cooder, Stevie Ray Vaughan, David Grohl, and Lionel Ritchie all do not read music. Prominent blind musicians such as Ray Charles, Stevie Wonder, Dianne Shurr, and Jose Feliciano have been successful without being able to read music.

Being able to "see" the correct notes, tempo, and so on, can accelerate learning unfamiliar music, although increasingly musicians can "see" how to play parts through on-line videos while also hearing how it should sound. If looking at music while playing, recording oneself is valuable, because the brain can focus on observing the notes more so than "hearing" what it how actually sounds.

SUMMARY

Music is a remedy, a tonic, orange juice for the ear. But for many of my neurological patients, music is even more — it can provide access, even when no medication can, to movement, to speech, to life. For them, music is not a luxury, but a necessity.

—Oliver Sacks

Music is a profound, available tool in clinical settings useful for enhancing mood, diminishing distress, widening one's experiences, and cultivating connections to others, including the clinician. Given that so many children are exposed to music and attempt playing an instrument during childhood, familiarity with musical benefits for the brain, routes to incorporate healthy musical routines into one's life, and practices to accomplish more in one's musical experiences provides another opportunity for clinicians to contribute to their patients' well-being.

REFERENCES

1. Sievers B, Polansky L, Casey M, et al. Music and movement share a dynamic structure that supports universal expressions of emotion. Proc Natl Acad Sci U S A 2013;110:70–5.
2. Koelsch S, Gunter TC, Friederici AD, et al. Brain indices of music processing: "nonmusicians" are musical. J Cogn Neurosci 2000;12:520–41.
3. Salimpoor VN, Benovoy M, Larcher K, et al. Anatomically distinct dopamine release during anticipation and experience of peak emotion to music. Nat Neurosci 2011;14:257–62.
4. Chen JL, Penhune VB, Zatorre RJ. Listening to musical rhythms recruits motor regions of the brain. Cereb Cortex 2008;18:2844–54.
5. Blood AJ, Zatorre RJ. Intensely pleasurable responses to music correlate with activity in brain regions implicated in reward and emotion. Proc Natl Acad Sci U S A 2001;98:11818–23.

6. Kraus N, Slater J, Thompson EC, et al. Auditory learning through active engagement with sound: biological impact of community music lessons in at-risk children. Front Neurosci 2014. https://doi.org/10.3389/fnins.2014.00351.
7. Hetland L. Listening to music enhances spatial-temporal reasoning: evidence for the "Mozart Effect". J Aesthetic Educ 2000;34:105–48.
8. Moreno S, Marques C, Santos A, et al. Musical training influences linguistic abilities in 8-year-old children: more evidence for brain plasticity. Cereb Cortex 2009; 19:712–23.
9. Schellenberg EG. Music lessons enhance IQ. Psychol Sci 2004;15:511–4.
10. Hudziak JJ, Albaugh MD, Ducharme S, et al. Music and cortical thickness development. J Am Acad Child Adolesc Psychiatry 2014;53(11):1153–61.
11. Rickard NS, Appleman P, James R, et al. Orchestrating life skills: the effect of increased school-based music classes on children's social competence and self-esteem. Int J Music Educ 2013;31:292–309.
12. Eerola PS, Eerola T. Extended music education enhances the quality of school life. Music Educ Res 2014;16(1):88–104.
13. Aleman X, Duryea S, Guerra N, et al. The effects of musical training on child development: a randomized trial of *El Sistema* in Venzuela. Prev Sci 2017;7: 865–78.
14. Choi A-N, Lee MS, Lee J-S. Group music intervention reduces aggression and improves self-esteem in children with highly aggressive behavior. Evid Based Complement Alternat Med 2010;7(2):213–7.
15. Beck RJ, Cesario TC, Yousefi A, et al. Choral singing, performance perception, and immune system changes in salivary immunoglobulin-a and cortisol. Music Percept 2000;18:87–106.
16. Ali SO, Peynircioglu ZF. Songs and emotions: are lyrics and melodies equal partners? Psychol Music 2006;34(4):511–34.
17. Litman RE, Farberow NL. Pop-rock music as precipitating cause in youth suicide. J Forensic Sci 1994;39:494–9.
18. Martinez-Molina N, Mas-Herrero E, Rodríguez-Fornells, et al. Neural correlates of specific musical anhedonia. Proc Natl Acad Sci U S A 2017;113(46):E7337–45.
19. Bonnerville-Roussy A, Rentfrow PJ, Xu MK, et al. Music through the ages: trends in musical engagement and preferences from adolescence through middle adulthood. J Personal Social Psychol 2013;105(4):703–17.
20. Frith S. Sound effects. Youth leisure and the politics of rock 'n'roll. New York: Pantheon; 1981.
21. Karageorghis CI, Priest DL. Music in the exercise domain: a review and synthesis (Part II). Int Rev Sport Exerc Psychol 2012;5:67–84.
22. American Psychological Association (2017). Stress in America: The State of Our Nation. Stress in America™ Survey.
23. Gallup Poll. Gallup organization reveals findings of "American attitudes toward making music survey. 2003 Available at: https://www.namm.org/news/press-releases/gallup-organization-reveals-findings-american-atti. Accessed December 18, 2018.
24. ABRMS (Associated Board of Royal Schools of Music). Making music: teaching, learning, and playing in the UK. 2014. Available at: https://gb.abrsm.org/en/making-music/4-the-statistics/. Accessed December 18, 2018.
25. Crickmore L. The measurement of aesthetic emotion in music. Front Psychol 2017. https://doi.org/10.3389/fpsyg.2017.00651.
26. Zentner M, Grandjean D, Scherer. Emotions evoked by the sound of music: characterization, classification, and measurement. Emotion 2008;8:494–521.

27. Nagel F, Kopiez R, Grewe O, et al. EMuJoy: software for continuous measurement of perceived emotions in music. Behav Res Methods 2007;39:283–90.
28. Seligman MEP. Authentic happiness. New York: Simon & Schuster; 2002.
29. Khalfa S, Bella SD, Roy M, et al. Effects of relaxing music on salivary cortisol level after psychological stress. Ann N Y Acad Sci 2003;999:374–6.
30. DeMarco J, Alexander JL, Nehrenz G, et al. The benefit of music for the reduction of stress and anxiety in patients undergoing elective cosmetic surgery. Music & Medicine 2012;4:44.
31. Dileo C, Bradt J. Music therapy: applications to stress management. In: Lehrer PM, editor. Principles and practice of stress management. Guilford Press; 2007. p. 519–44.
32. Bringman H, Giesecke K, Thome A, et al. Relaxing music as pre-medication before surgery; a randomized controlled trial. Acta Anaesthesiol Scand 2009; 53:759–64.
33. Bradt J, Dileo C, Shim M (2013). Music interventions for preoperative anxiety. Cochrane Database Syst Rev 6:CD006908.
34. Ziv N, Chaim AB, Itamar O. The effect of positive music and dispositional hope on state hope and affect. Psychol Music 2011;38:3–17.
35. Sloboda JA, Juslin PN. Psychological perspectives on music and emotion. In: Juslin PN, Sloboda JA, editors. Music and emotion: theory and research. Oxford University Press; 2001. p. 71–104.
36. Huron D. Why is sad music pleasurable? A possible role for prolactin. Musicae Scientiae 2011;15(2):146–58.
37. Good M, Anderson GC, Ahn S, et al. Relaxation and music reduce pain following intestinal surgery. Res Nurs Health 2002;28:240–51.
38. Strachan DL. The space between the notes: the effects of background music on student focus. Retrieved from Sophia, the St. Catherine University repository website. 2015. Available at: https://sophia.stkate.edu/maed/118. Accessed December 18, 2018.
39. Anderson S, Hencke J, McLaughlin M, et al. Using background music to enhance memory and improve learning. ERIC; 2000. ED437663.
40. Langan K, Sachs DE. Opening Pandora's stream: piping music into the information literacy classroom. Publ Serv Q 2013;9(2). https://doi.org/10.1080/15228959. 2013.785876.
41. Dolegui AS. The impact of listening to music on cognitive performance. Inquiries Journal 2013;50(9):1–21.
42. Thompson WF, Schellenberg EG, Letnic AK (2012). Fast and loud background music disrupts reading comprehension. Psychology of Music 40700-708.
43. Tze-Ming Chou P. Attention drainage effect: how background music effects concentration in Taiwanese college students. J Schol Teach Learn 2011;10:36–46.
44. Pring L, Walker J. The effects of unvocalized music on short-term memory. Curr Psychol 1994;13:165–71.
45. Huron D. Is music an evolutionary adaptation? Ann N Y Acad Sci 2001;930: 43–61.
46. Levitin DJ. The world in six songs: how the musical brain created human nature. New York: Plume/Penguin; 2009.
47. Thompson RL, Larson R. Social context and the subjective experience of different types of rock music. J Youth Adolesc 1995;24:731–44.
48. Grape C, Sandren M, Hansson LO, et al. Does singing promote well-being? An empirical study of professional and amateur singers during a singing lesson. Integr Physiol Behav Sci 2003;38:65–74.

49. Guéguen N, Jacob C, Lamy L. Love is in the air: effects of songs with romantic lyrics on compliance with a courtship request. Psychol Music 2010;38:303–7.
50. Juslin PN, Laukka P. Communication of emotions in vocal expression and music performance: different channels, same code? Psychol Bull 2003;129:770–814.
51. Reimer B. Why do humans value music? Presented at the Music Educators National Conference, Reston, VA. 2000. Available at: https://nafme.org/wp-content/files/2015/12/6-WhyDoHumansValueMusic-by-Bennett-Reimer.pdf. Accessed December 18, 2018.
52. Duke R, Simmons A, Cash C. It's not how much: it's how. J Res Music Educ 2009; 56:310–21.

Applying Mindfulness-Based Practices in Child Psychiatry

Erin T. Mathis, PhD[a], Elizabeth Dente, BA[b],
Matthew G. Biel, MD, MSc[c,d],*

KEYWORDS

- Mindfulness • Meditation • MBSR • Self-regulation

KEY POINTS

- Mindfulness-based interventions for adults, children, and families have a growing evidence base for treatment of a range of clinical concerns.
- Emerging research suggest that mindfulness-based interventions have their effect through impact on attentional processes and emotional regulation.
- Practicing child and adolescent psychiatrists should familiarize themselves with the basics of mindfulness-based interventions, refer children and families to receive these services when concerns about self-regulation are prominent, and should consider integrating mindfulness into their own clinical practices.

HISTORICAL CONTEXT AND DEFINITION OF MINDFULNESS AND MINDFULNESS MEDITATION

Mindfulness practices are grounded in the belief that human suffering exists because we tend not to appreciate or accept the impermanent nature of our experiences. We have a natural tendency to attempt to extend or intensify pleasant experiences and minimize or stop unpleasant experiences. Buddhist traditions identify this desire to change our current experiences as a source of distress, and they teach that relief can be found through acceptance of the present moment. This capacity to accept sensations, thoughts, and feelings in the present moment, without trying to change

Disclosure Statement: none.
[a] Department of Psychiatry, Center for Child and Human Development, Georgetown University Medical Center, 3300 Whitehaven Street Northwest, Washington, DC 20007, USA; [b] Georgetown University School of Medicine, 3900 Reservoir Road Northwest, Washington, DC 20057, USA; [c] Department of Psychiatry, Medstar Georgetown University Hospital, Georgetown University Medical Center, Georgetown University, 2115 Wisconsin Avenue Northwest, Washington, DC 20007, USA; [d] Department of Pediatrics, Medstar Georgetown University Hospital, 2115 Wisconsin Avenue NW, Washington, DC 20007, USA
* Corresponding author. Department of Psychiatry, Medstar Georgetown University Hospital, 2115 Wisconsin Avenue NW, Washington, DC 20007.
E-mail address: mgb33@georgetown.edu

them, is cultivated in the Buddhist tradition through meditation practices, including mindfulness meditation.

Although mindfulness has been part of the Buddhist tradition for thousands of years, more recently secular versions of this approach have been developed to address health and well-being. Mindfulness-based approaches have been applied in clinical settings for more than 40 years in North America. Kabat-Zinn[1,2] at the University of Massachusetts was an early leader of these efforts and defined mindfulness as paying attention to the present moment, on purpose and without judgment. Kabat-Zinn and colleagues[3,4] created mindfulness training exercises designed to practice sustaining attention in the present moment in an open and receptive state, to cultivate awareness of the relation between thoughts, emotions and bodily sensations, and to accept them without the evaluation of being good or bad. These strategies led to development in the late 1970s of an intervention program called Mindfulness-Based Stress Reduction (MBSR). MBSR was created for patients with chronic severe medical illnesses and was designed as a class that met weekly over 8 weeks and introduced patients to fundamental concepts and basic practices of mindful awareness, mindful breathing, mindfulness meditation, mindful movement, and cultivation of compassion and lovingkindness.[3,4] See **Box 1** for a summary of the key components of clinical applications of mindfulness practices.

The application of MBSR to clinical populations has grown enormously in subsequent decades, with many dozens of clinical trials producing consistent and replicated findings of clinically meaningful reductions in medical and psychological symptoms across a range of physical and mental health conditions, both during the 8-week intervention and for up to 4 years postintervention. Studies demonstrating clinically significant responses to the intervention have included MBSR for adults with cardiac conditions, chronic pain, autoimmune conditions, chronic gastrointestinal conditions, and obesity. Within psychiatry, studies suggest significant clinical benefit of MBSR for patients with depression, anxiety disorders, eating disorders, sleep disorders, and addiction.[5–8]

As dissemination of MBSR and MBSR-inspired approaches has grown, the original creators of the intervention have been supportive of adaptations of MBSR while emphasizing the need to maintain several standards of practice, including an emphasis on daily practice, an educational rather than therapeutic approach to classes, and medically heterogeneous groups that emphasize shared positive traits among class members rather than shared diagnoses or deficits.[2] In addition to numerous versions of MBSR, new clinical interventions based in mindfulness-based approaches have been developed, many specifically targeting psychiatric conditions and primarily designed for adult patients.

Box 1
Key components of clinical applications of mindfulness practices

Attention: actively attending to thoughts, feelings, and sensations

Intention: purposeful focus

Present moment: emphasis on moment-by-moment experiences in the "here and now"

Nonjudgment: acceptance of thoughts, feelings, and sensations without criticism

Attitude: openness and curiosity toward thoughts, feelings, and sensations

Compassion: actively cultivating feelings of kindness and acceptance toward self and others

Data from Kabat-Zinn J. Mindfulness meditation: what it is, what it isn't, and its role in health care and medicine. In: Haruki Y, Ishii Y, Suzuki M, editors. Comparative and psychological study on meditation. Delft (Netherlands): Eburon; 1996; and Baer RA. Mindfulness training as a clinical intervention: a conceptual and empirical review. Clin Psychol Sci Pract 2003;10(2):125–43.

Mindfulness-Based Cognitive Therapy (MBCT) combines mindfulness-based approaches developed in MBSR with cognitive strategies from traditional cognitive psychotherapy to address persistent and recurrent depressive symptoms in adults with recurrent major depression.[9] MBCT has demonstrated efficacy in preventing relapse in these patients.[10] Mindfulness strategies are also used as part of a broader suite of skills-based approaches in Dialectical Behavioral Therapy (DBT) and Acceptance and Commitment Therapy (ACT).[7,11,12] Most mindfulness-based interventions share several core characteristics, including brief duration (typically 16 weeks or fewer), delivery in group-based settings, and training in meditation practices to bring awareness to the present moment without judgment.[13]

MINDFULNESS-BASED INTERVENTIONS WITH CHILDREN, ADOLESCENTS, PARENTS, AND TEACHERS

Emerging research on mindfulness-based intervention strategies with children and adolescents has indicated a range of benefits, including improvements in attention control, behavior regulation, and emotion regulation, as well as a reduction in clinical symptoms, such as depression, anxiety, and disruptive behaviors.[14–16] Findings from a range of studies suggest that mindfulness-based interventions with children and adolescents have the potential for positive outcomes when used both at the universal level for prevention and promotion of well-being, as well as at a targeted level to improve symptoms in clinical populations.

Mindfulness training has the potential to facilitate the healthy development of self-regulation in children.[17] In particular, mindfulness practice provides children and adolescents with multiple opportunities to become consciously aware of their thoughts and feelings. This awareness may allow youth to thoughtfully respond in situations rather than react impulsively or engage in harmful behaviors. Observing the present moment and recognizing one's thoughts, emotions, and sensations can lead to increased capacity for emotional regulation and reduced susceptibility to feeling overwhelmed or preoccupied with ruminative thoughts.[18–20]

Mindfulness-based interventions are increasingly being used in the treatment of mental health symptoms in children and adolescents. Several studies have examined training in mindfulness meditation with clinical populations, including children and/or adolescents with attention-deficit/hyperactivity disorder, anxiety, and disruptive behavior disorders.[21,22] These studies report improvements in outcomes such as anxiety symptoms and behavior problems.[23,24]

Some specific mindfulness-based interventions that were previously developed for adults in the clinical setting have been adapted and tested with children and adolescents. For example, Biegel and colleagues[14] adapted MBSR for teens to specifically focus on interpersonal challenges and related stress that is common in adolescence. The sessions and mindfulness practice exercises were shorter than in the traditional MBSR program and the day-long retreat was replaced with weekly check-ins to provide additional support and to help generalize the MBSR skills to daily life.[14] Results from their randomized controlled trial for adolescents ages 14 to 18 showed that adolescents who participated in the adapted MBSR program reported a reduction in anxiety and depression symptoms as well as somatic distress. Participants also reported an increase in self-esteem and sleep quality. At 3-month follow-up, participants showed the greatest improvement in diagnosis (45% of the MBSR group showed diagnostic change, which was most pronounced in the mood disorder group, compared with almost no change in the control group) and had significant increases in clinician-rated global assessment of functioning scores.

MBCT-C is an adaptation of MBCT for children and has been evaluated for children ages 9 to 13 years.[23,25] MBCT-C was adapted to be more developmentally appropriate for younger children, including the following:

1. Decreasing the length of mindfulness practices and the length of the sessions, while also focusing more on repetition of content to allow for more practice
2. Focusing more on sensory experiences rather than more abstract concepts, such as internal experiences and thoughts
3. Including parents in the intervention to support generalization to children's daily life

Results from a randomized controlled trial showed that children who participated in MBCT-C had fewer attention problems than waitlist control. The reduction in attention problems accounted for 46% of the variance of changes in behavior problems and improvements in attention were maintained at 3-month follow-up. In addition, there was a significant reduction in anxiety symptoms and behavior problems for children who entered the program with clinically elevated level of anxiety, suggesting that MBCT-C might be particularly effective with this population. MBCT-C has also been adapted and manualized specifically for children who experience anxiety.[26]

Several reviews have summarized evidence on the use of mindfulness with children and adolescents in clinical practice. Simkin and Black[27] provide a comprehensive overview of the literature organized by specific intervention method and clinical diagnosis targeted in each study. Zoogman and colleagues[28] published the first meta-analysis on mindfulness-based interventions for children and adolescents younger than 18 using studies up to 2011. The investigators found an overall positive effect of mindfulness interventions for children and adolescents over active control comparisons with a small to moderate effect size. Larger effect sizes were found specifically for psychological symptoms compared with other outcome types and for clinical populations compared with nonclinical populations, providing further support for the utility of mindfulness-based interventions for youth with impairing emotional and behavioral symptomatology. Kallapiran and colleagues[29] published a meta-analysis of mindfulness-based interventions on clinical and nonclinical samples of children and adolescents using studies up to 2014. The investigators grouped MBSR and MBCT studies together, citing that the 2 interventions use similar approaches and teach similar techniques, and found that the MBSR/MBCT group was more effective in improving stress, anxiety and depression compared with the nonactive, nonclinical control group. In clinical populations, ACT was equally as effective in the management of anxiety, depression, and overall quality of life compared with active treatment through other modalities. The investigators combined all other groups (eg, yoga, other meditation practices) into a third group and found that they were more effective in improving stress and anxiety, but not depression, as compared with the nonactive, nonclinical control group.

A large segment of the literature examining mindfulness-based interventions with children and adolescents focuses on using mindfulness with nonclinical populations in universal school settings, and includes programs such as Learning to BREATHE,[30,31] Inner Kids,[32] MindUP,[33] and Master Mind.[34] Universal mindfulness programs focus on common stressors rather than specific problems or pathologies. Using a strengths-based approach, these programs address an entire classroom or an entire school and seek to normalize stress and worry as everyday experiences faced by most children. Despite high prevalence rates of anxiety and depression among youth, many children and parents do not access clinical intervention for mental health concerns in outpatient settings. Universal mindfulness interventions in the school setting offers a way to promote emotional and behavioral health in all students, and to reach students with clinical concerns who otherwise might not access support or treatment.

For example, Learning to BREATHE was developed for adolescents to improve emotion regulation and attention control and to reduce stress, and was designed to be delivered in the classroom setting. The program was evaluated in 2 nonrandomized trials.[30,31] In the first trial, compared with controls, participants reported significant decreases in negative affect and increases in feelings of calmness, relaxation and self-acceptance, as well as improvements in emotion regulation. In a follow-up trial, Metz and colleagues[31] found that participants reported statistically significant decreased levels of perceived stress and psychosomatic symptoms and higher levels of emotion regulation, including emotional awareness, access to regulation strategies, and emotional clarity, indicating that the program may be an effective intervention for the development of social-emotional learning skills.

The Master Mind program was developed to promote healthy decision making and support self-regulation. The program includes core mindfulness practices, including mindful breathing, mindful meditation, mindful movement, real-world applications, and daily practices. The program was evaluated in a small randomized controlled trial using a waitlist control, and demonstrated significant improvements for both boys and girls in executive function skills as well as significant reductions in aggression and social problems.[34] There was also a significant improvement in self-control abilities in boys and a reduction in anxiety symptoms in girls.

MINDFULNESS WITH TEACHERS AND PARENTS

Teaching is a cognitively, emotionally, and attentionally demanding profession that includes pressing demands and performance expectations, often leading to increased levels of stress among teachers.[35] High stress levels can lead to frequent negative emotions that can impair a teacher's cognitive functioning and well-being, ultimately creating a negative impact on instruction quality.[36] High levels of stress are associated with decreases in motivation and overall teaching efficacy.[37] Chronic stress can lead to burnout, work-related fatigue, depression, and anxiety over time.[38,39] In the same way that stress and distress is transmitted between family members, a teacher's stress levels can also impact the children in the classroom through "passive exposure," whereby teachers in a state of heightened stress model poor coping strategies and are harsh with students.[40]

Mindfulness is a promising approach to mitigate stress and improve teachers' sense of well-being. Teachers who practice mindfulness experience less stress, are better able to regulate their attention and emotions, and report increased professional self-efficacy.[37] For example, the Cultivating Awareness and Resilience in Education (CARE) program is a mindfulness program for teachers that has a growing evidence base. CARE primarily focuses on 3 components: emotional skills instruction, mindfulness and stress reduction, and listening and compassion exercises.[41] These components are taught to teachers through a combination of direct instruction, interactive activities, discussions, and reflection at home, all designed to promote mindfulness and emotional awareness and regulation.[42] CARE has been found effective in a variety of studies in different settings and has shown improvements in teachers' emotion regulation, mindfulness, psychological distress, and sense of time pressure.[43–45] The authors have also found an improvement in classroom climate, specifically the emotional support in the classroom.[43] The growing literature on mindfulness with teachers suggests that this is a promising approach for promoting teachers' social-emotional competence, sense of well-being and the quality of their classroom climate.

Mindful parenting has been defined as paying attention to the present moment, and expressing compassion, acceptance, and kindness toward children during the parenting process.[46] Mindfulness encourages parents to be thoughtful when making parenting decisions, and involves processes such as focused attention and listening, self-regulation in the parent-child relationship, acceptance, emotional awareness, and compassion for self and child.[47,48] Mindful parenting has been shown to benefit both parents and children, fostering positive parent-youth interactions and increasing parental presence, compassion, and acceptance, while reducing stress for both parents and children.[47,49–51] Mindful parenting skills promote secure attachments and enhance children's emotion regulation skills, thereby reducing the likelihood of children developing emotional symptoms, hyperactivity, and peer problems.[52] Mindful parenting programs, when combined with other positive parenting skills instruction, also have been shown to decrease the risk of child abuse and increase family functioning.[51]

PROPOSED MECHANISMS OF MINDFULNESS-BASED INTERVENTIONS

What are the mechanisms by which mindfulness-based approaches generate positive clinical impact on such a wide range of patient populations? How might these proposed mechanisms illuminate the role for mindfulness-based interventions in the clinical care of children, adolescents, and families, as well as for more universal emotional and behavioral health promotion? Recent evidence supports diverse psychological and physiologic impact of these practices.

One of the central drivers of change with mindfulness practices may occur through impact on attentional processes.[53,54] Attentional control, the capacity to direct attention to relevant external stimuli and internal emotional and physical processes, and to allocate limited attentional resources to the most salient information and cognitive tasks, is a crucial component of healthy emotional and behavioral functioning. Key components of mindfulness training, including focusing on the present moment and identifying and accepting mental and emotional states without judgment, can be conceptualized as attentional tasks that significantly involve several key brain regions, including the insula and the right temporo-parietal junction. Both areas are implicated in attentional control and show enhanced activity in experienced meditators.[55–57] The insula in particular is involved in interoception, the capacity for perceiving internal physical and mental states that may correlate to the focused self-perception and self-awareness cultivated in mindfulness practice.[56]

Emotional regulation, the capacity to initiate, adjust, and control emotions, moods, and affects in response to experiences and sensations, is a key factor in emotional and behavioral well-being throughout the life span. Challenges or deficits in emotional regulation skills are often implicated in mood, anxiety, and personality disorders, and are likely relevant in interpersonal difficulties, including parent-child interactions. Emerging evidence suggests that mindfulness practice may build emotional regulation skills, perhaps through enhanced attentional control and emotional acceptance.[58] Mindfulness may also improve information processing in emotionally challenging situations by impacting the allocation of attentional resources to emotional stimuli.[59,60]

In addition to accumulating evidence of the impact of mindfulness practice on attentional processes and emotional regulation, recent studies suggest observable physiologic buffering of stress responses in mindful individuals. In one noteworthy study, researchers investigated correlations between distressed emotional state and physiologic response in individuals with high and low trait levels of mindfulness. Using the cortisol awakening response as a measure of stress response in the setting of emotional distress, they found that individuals with low levels of mindfulness show heightened cortisol response to emotional distress, whereas individuals with high levels of mindfulness showed no increase in cortisol response when emotionally distressed. The investigators propose that the mindful ability to describe and accept distressing emotional events can buffer the impact of distressing emotional events on physiologic stress response.[61] Given the well-described association between sustained elevated cortisol levels and negative outcomes in mental and physical health, this buffering effect suggests an important potential role for mindfulness training, perhaps particularly in settings of high rates of adversity or chronic stress.

A recent review of neurophysiological investigations of mindfulness practitioners suggests that the state of relaxed alertness that individuals achieve while meditating may be correlated with increased alpha and theta synchronization and power on electroencephalogram in both novice and experienced meditators and in both healthy and clinical populations.[62] Increased alpha synchronization, in particular, correlates with strengthening of "inward-directed" attention and improved performance on attentional tasks, providing electrophysiological support for the positive impact of meditation on attentional systems.[62] One recent study suggests that mindful breathing exercises may enhance attentional engagement and self-monitoring, with novice meditator participants showing increased alpha power during breathing exercises and enhanced capacity for self-monitoring and error-correction during a subsequent cognitive task.[63] These and other studies in a growing body of literature support the neurophysiological impact of meditation, and this evidence suggests that inexperienced meditators and both healthy and clinically impaired populations may experience positive impact on attentional capacities with these practices.

In summary, recent studies suggest that the practice of mindfulness supports the development of important attentional skills, specifically the capacities to attend to internal physical and emotional states, to observe and describe these states without judgment, and to maintain this self-awareness and lack of reactivity during activities and experiences. These capacities seem to contribute to positive changes in psychological well-being and improved emotional and behavioral self-regulation.[57] As self-regulation is so commonly a core concern for children and families presenting for psychiatric consultation, the relevance of these intervention strategies in clinical practice is increasingly evident.

MINDFULNESS-BASED PRACTICES IN CLINICAL PRACTICE OF CHILD AND ADOLESCENT PSYCHIATRY

The preceding sections of this article outlined the historical development, clinical evolution, and expanding scientific bases supporting the use of mindfulness to bolster emotional and behavioral well-being. Although MBSR was once the primary mode of introducing patients to mindfulness, the creation of a range of other clinical protocols, such as MBCT, DBT, and ACT, for both adults and youth, as well as the integration of mindfulness principles and practices into classroom instruction, family-focused and parent-focused interventions, and group and individual psychotherapies, has considerably broadened ways in which children and families may be introduced to mindfulness. How can practicing child psychiatrists begin to incorporate mindfulness-based strategies into their clinical work, and include mindfulness interventions in their treatment planning?

The first step for many providers will be to identify resources offering mindfulness-based interventions within their own practice settings, affiliated clinical entities, and broader communities. Many hospital-based outpatient clinics, community mental health clinics, and group practices have begun to offer mindfulness-based clinical services to both adult and child patients, and child psychiatrists can begin to establish referral relationships with these practices. As described previously, many mindfulness-based interventions are time-limited and skills-based, and as a result these programs may be more accessible than more open-ended clinical programs that are often unable to accept new referrals. Child psychiatrists have the opportunity to meet and assess both children and parents and caregivers during evaluation and care and may consider mindfulness-based interventions to be relevant strategies to support self-regulation skills in one or more family members' own emotional and behavioral health, as well as to specifically address parenting challenges. In addition, many schools ranging from early childhood education through high school offer mindfulness-based supports to students, and collaboration with school staff to reinforce implementation of these strategies can be useful.

Child psychiatrists in leadership positions in clinical settings might consider initiating mindfulness-based clinical programs where none exist. Increasing public interest in mindfulness and meditation means that these programs are often eagerly received when offered. The focus on building "skills for life" through mindfulness training is appealing to many adults and children, and this framing may alleviate stigma associated with seeking mental health care for some families. Public and private insurance coverage for mindfulness-based interventions varies according to practice location, specific modality of treatment, and other factors, and should be investigated before initiating services.

Training is widely available for clinicians interested in delivering established evidence-based models of care, including MBSR, MBCT, DBT, and ACT for adults and youth, as well as mindfulness-based parenting training. Many child psychiatrists have been trained in these programs and go on to provide direct clinical care with these modalities, and child psychiatrists leading inpatient, intensive outpatient, outpatient, and school-based clinical services can integrate mindfulness-based programs into these treatment settings. Clinical staff, including psychologists, social workers, licensed counselors and therapists, and nurses and nurse practitioners, often have pursued training in these modalities and can lead and co-lead individual and group-based interventions. Many child mental health clinicians have begun to include one or more brief mindfulness exercises into treatment visits as a routine aspect of care, and to prescribe regular practice of these exercises between visits. A brief listing of mindfulness-based practices that can be incorporated into routine clinical encounters in any clinical setting is included in **Table 1**, together with an estimated time require for the practice and clinical factors to consider in choosing among practices.

Mindfulness has begun to significantly impact the practice of mental health care for both adults and children beyond the parameters of specific evidence-based treatment

Table 1
Example mindfulness practices to incorporate into routine clinical encounters

Mindfulness Practice	Time Required, min	Clinical Target
Diaphragmatic breathing ("belly breathing")	1–2	Anxiety and mood regulation, attention, trauma
Body scan	2–3	Anxiety, trauma
Brief mindful movement practice	2–3	Hyperactivity, attention, trauma
Brief mindfulness meditation	3–5	Anxiety and mood regulation, attention, trauma
Brief lovingkindness meditation	3–5 min	Mood regulation, depression, trauma

programs. Psychotherapy training in a variety of disciplines, including child and adolescent psychiatry, increasingly includes at least brief introductions to the role of mindfulness in emotional and behavioral well-being, as well as in the treatment of mental illness. Continuing education and professional development opportunities for practicing psychiatrists may feature introductory training in the use of mindfulness-based approaches in routine clinical practice. As evidence for the impact of mindfulness in keeping adults and children well, and in restoring to good emotional and behavioral health those who are struggling with self-regulation difficulties and other mental health symptoms, practicing clinicians will increasingly be drawn to familiarizing themselves with these approaches and to introducing basic mindfulness practices into routine clinical care. Teaching young people and the adults who care for them to pay attention to their thoughts and feelings, on purpose and without judgment, and to develop daily habits and practices that reinforce these abilities, is part of a growing suite of interventions that are relevant for maintaining emotional and behavioral well-being across the life course.

REFERENCES

1. Kabat-Zinn J. Full catastrophe living: using the wisdom of your body and mind to face stress, pain, and illness. New York: Dell Publishing; 1990.
2. Kabat-Zinn J. Mindfulness meditation: what it is, what it isn't, and its role in health care and medicine. In: Haruki Y, Ishii Y, Suzuki M, editors. Comparative and psychological study on meditation. Delft, Netherlands: Eburon; 1996. p. 161–9.
3. Kabat-Zinn J. An outpatient program in behavioral medicine for chronic pain patients based on the practice of mindfulness meditation: theoretical considerations and preliminary results. Gen Hosp Psychiatry 1982;4(1):33–47.
4. Kabat-Zinn J, Lipworth L, Burney R, et al. Four-year follow-up of a meditation-based program for the self-regulation of chronic pain: treatment outcomes and compliance. Clin J Pain 1987;3(1):60.
5. Baer RA. Mindfulness training as a clinical intervention: a conceptual and empirical review. Clin Psychol Sci Pract 2003;10(2):125–43.
6. de Vibe M, Solhaug I, Tyssen R, et al. Mindfulness training for stress management: a randomised controlled study of medical and psychology students. BMC Med Educ 2013;13(1):107.
7. Grossman P, Niemann L, Schmidt S, et al. Mindfulness-based stress reduction and health benefits: a meta-analysis. J Psychosom Res 2004;57:35–43.
8. Hofmann SG, Sawyer AT, Witt AA, et al. The effect of mindfulness-based therapy on anxiety and depression: a meta-analytic review. J Consult Clin Psychol 2010; 78(2):169.
9. Segal ZV, Williams JMG, Teasdale JD. Mindfulness-based cognitive therapy for depression: a new approach to preventing relapse. New York: The Guilford Press; 2002.
10. Kuyken W, Byford S, Taylor RS, et al. Mindfulness based cognitive therapy to prevent relapse in recurrent depression. J Consult Clin Psychol 2008;76(6):966–78.
11. Linehan MM. Cognitive behavioral therapy of borderline personality disorder, vol. 51. New York: Guilford Press; 1993.
12. Hayes L, Boyd CP, Sewell J. Acceptance and commitment therapy for the treatment of adolescent depression: a pilot study in a psychiatric outpatient setting. Mindfulness 2011;2:86–94.

13. Strauss C, Cavanagh K, Oliver A, et al. Mindfulness-based interventions for people diagnosed with a current episode of an anxiety or depressive disorder: a meta-analysis of randomised controlled trials. PLoS One 2014;9(4):e96110.

14. Biegel GM, Brown KW, Shapiro SL, et al. Mindfulness-based stress reduction for the treatment of adolescent psychiatric outpatients: a randomized clinical trial. J Consult Clin Psychol 2009;77(5):855.

15. Broderick PC, Metz S. Learning to BREATHE: a pilot trial of a mindfulness curriculum for adolescents. Adv Sch Ment Health Promot 2009;2:35–46.

16. Schonert-Reichl KA, Lawlor MS. The effects of a mindfulness-based education program on pre- and early adolescents' well-being and social and emotional competence. Mindfulness 2010;1(3):137–51.

17. Zelazo P, Lyons KE. The potential benefits of mindfulness training in early childhood: a developmental social cognitive neuroscience perspective. Child Dev Perspect 2012;6(2):154–60.

18. Jain S, Shapiro SL, Swanick S, et al. A randomized controlled trial of mindfulness meditation versus relaxation training: effects on distress, positive states of mind, rumination, and distraction. Ann Behav Med 2007;33:11–21.

19. Eberth J, Sedlmeier P. The effects of mindfulness meditation: a meta-analysis. Mindfulness 2012;3:174–89.

20. Jimenez SS, Niles BL, Park CL. A mindfulness model of affect regulation and depressive symptoms: positive emotions, mood regulation expectancies, and self-acceptance as regulatory mechanisms. Pers Indiv Differ 2010;49:645–50.

21. Black DS. Mindfulness training for children and adolescents. Handbook of Mindfulness: Theory, Research, and Practice 2015;283:246–63.

22. Burke CA. Mindfulness-based approaches with children and adolescents: a preliminary review of current research in an emergent field. J Child Fam Stud 2010; 19(2):133–44.

23. Semple R, Lee J, Rosa D, et al. A randomized trial of mindfulness-based cognitive therapy for children: promoting mindful attention to enhance social-emotional resiliency in children. J Child Fam Stud 2010;19(2):218–29.

24. Van de Weijer-Bergsma E, Formsma AR, de Bruin EI, et al. The effectiveness of mindfulness training on behavioral problems and attentional functioning in adolescents with ADHD. J Child Fam Stud 2012;21(5):775–87.

25. Lee J, Semple RJ, Rosa D, et al. Mindfulness-based cognitive therapy for children: results of a pilot study. J Cognit Psychother 2008;22(1):15.

26. Semple RJ, Lee J. Mindfulness-based cognitive therapy for anxious children: a manual for treating childhood anxiety. Oakland (CA): New Harbinger Publications, Inc; 2011.

27. Simkin DR, Black NB. Meditation and mindfulness in clinical practice. Child Adolesc Psychiatr Clin 2014;23(3):487–534.

28. Zoogman S, Goldberg SB, Hoyt WT, et al. Mindfulness interventions with youth: a meta-analysis. Mindfulness 2014;6(2):290–302.

29. Kallapiran K, Koo S, Kirubakaran R, et al. Effectiveness of mindfulness in improving mental health symptoms of children and adolescents: a meta-analysis. Child Adolesc Ment Health 2015;20(4):182–94.

30. Broderick PC. Learning to BREATHE: a mindfulness curriculum for adolescents to cultivate emotion regulation, attention, and performance. Oakland (CA): New Harbinger; 2013.

31. Metz SM, Frank JF, Reibel D, et al. The effectiveness of the Learning to BREATHE program on adolescent emotion regulation. Res Hum Dev 2013;10(3):252–72.

32. Flook L, Smalley SL, Kitil MJ, et al. Effects of mindful awareness practices on executive functions in elementary school children. J Appl Sch Psychol 2010;26(1): 70–95.

33. Schonert-Reichl KA, Oberle E, Lawlor MS, et al. Enhancing cognitive and social-emotional development through a simple-to-administer mindfulness-based school program for elementary school children: a randomized controlled trial. Dev Psychol 2015;51(1):52.

34. Parker AE, Kupersmidt JB, Mathis ET, et al. The impact of mindfulness education on elementary school students: evaluation of the Master Mind program. Adv Sch Ment Health Promot 2014;7(3):184–204.

35. Dworkin AG, Tobe PF. The effects of standards based school accountability on teacher burnout and trust relationships: a longitudinal analysis. In: VanMaele D, Forsyth P, Van Houtte M, editors. Trust and school life. Dordrecht (Netherlands): Springer; 2014. p. 121–43.

36. Carson R, Weiss H, Templin T. Ecological momentary assessment: a research method for studying the daily lives of teachers. Int J Res Meth Educ 2010; 33(2):165–82.

37. Kavanagh DJ, Bower G. Mood and self-efficacy: impact of joy and sadness on perceived capabilities. Cognit Ther Res 1985;9:507–25.

38. Emerson LM, Leyland A, Hudson K, et al. Teaching mindfulness to teachers: a systematic review and narrative synthesis. Mindfulness 2017;8(5):1136–49.

39. Tsouloupas CN, Carson RL, Matthews R, et al. Exploring the association between teachers' perceived student misbehaviour and emotional exhaustion: the importance of teacher efficacy beliefs and emotion regulation. Educ Psychol 2010; 30(2):173–89.

40. Milkie MA, Warner CH. Classroom learning environments and the mental health of first grade children. J Health Soc Behav 2011;52(1):4–22.

41. Jennings PA. CARE for teachers: a mindfulness-based approach to promoting teachers' social and emotional competence and well-being. In: Schonert-Reichl K, Roeser R, editors. Handbook of mindfulness in education. New York: Springer; 2016. p. 133–48.

42. Jennings PA, Snowberg KE, Coccia MA, et al. Improving classroom learning environments by cultivating awareness and resilience in education (CARE): results of two pilot studies. The Journal of Classroom Interaction 2011;37–48.

43. Jennings PA, Brown JL, Frank JL, et al. Impacts of the CARE for Teachers program on teachers' social and emotional competence and classroom interactions. J Educ Psychol 2017;109(7):1010.

44. Jennings PA, Frank JL, Snowberg KE, et al. Improving classroom learning environments by Cultivating Awareness and Resilience in Education (CARE): results of a randomized controlled trial. Sch Psychol Q 2013;28(4):374.

45. Schussler DL, Jennings PA, Sharp JE, et al. Improving teacher awareness and well-being through CARE: a qualitative analysis of the underlying mechanisms. Mindfulness 2016;7(1):130–42.

46. Kabat-Zinn M, Kabat-Zinn J. Everyday blessings: the inner work of mindful parenting. New York: Hyperion; 1997.

47. Campbell K, Thoburn JW, Leonard HD. The mediating effects of stress on the relationship between mindfulness and parental responsiveness. Couple Family Psychol 2017;6(1):48–59.

48. Duncan LG, Coatsworth JD, Greenberg MT. A model of mindful parenting: implications for parent–child relationships and prevention research. Clin Child Fam Psychol Rev 2009;12(3):255–70.

49. Burns B, Haynes L, Bauer A, et al. Strengthening children's resilience through parenting: a pilot study. Ther Communities 2013;34(4):121–31.

50. Coatsworth JD, Duncan LG, Greenberg MT, et al. Changing parent's mindfulness, child management skills and relationship quality with their youth: results from a randomized pilot intervention trial. J Child Fam Stud 2010;19(2):203–17.

51. Coatsworth JD, Duncan LG, Nix RL, et al. Integrating mindfulness with parent training: effects of the mindfulness-enhanced strengthening families program. Dev Psychol 2015;51(1):26.

52. Siu AF, Ma Y, Chui FW. Maternal mindfulness and child social behavior: the mediating role of the mother-child relationship. Mindfulness 2016;7(3):577–83.

53. Bishop S. What do we really know about mindfulness-based stress reduction? Psychosom Med 2002;64:71–84.

54. Jha A, Krompinger J, Baime M. Mindfulness training modifies subsystems of attention. Cogn Affect Behav Neurosci 2007;7:109–19.

55. Gundel F, von Spee J, Schneider S, et al. Meditation and the brain—neuronal correlates of mindfulness as assessed with near-infrared spectroscopy. Psychiatry Res Neuroimaging 2018;271:24–33.

56. Young KS, van der Velden AM, Craske MG, et al. The impact of mindfulness-based interventions on brain activity: a systematic review of functional magnetic resonance imaging studies. Neurosci Biobehav Rev 2017;84:424–33.

57. Baer RA. Self-focused attention and mechanisms of change in mindfulness-based treatment. Cogn Behav Ther 2009;38(Supp 1):15–20.

58. Grecucci A, DePisapia N, Thero DK, et al. Baseline and strategic effects behind mindful emotion regulation: behavioral and physiological investigation. PLoS One 2015;10(1):e00116541.

59. Fan Y, Tang YY, Tang R, et al. Time course of conflict processing modulated by brief meditation training. Front Psychol 2015;6:911.

60. Eddy MD, Brunyé TT, Tower-Richardi S, et al. The effect of a brief mindfulness induction on processing of emotional images: an ERP study. Front Psychol 2015;6:1391.

61. Daubenmier J, Hayden D, Chang V, et al. It's not what you think, it's how you relate to it: dispositional mindfulness moderates the relationship between psychological distress and the cortisol awakening response. Psychoneuroendocrinology 2014;48:11–8.

62. Lomas T, Ivtzan I, Fu CH. A systematic review of the neurophysiology of mindfulness on EEG oscillations. Neurosci Biobehav Rev 2015;57:401–10.

63. Bing-Canar H, Pizzuto J, Compton RJ. Mindfulness-of-breathing exercise modulates EEG alpha activity during cognitive performance. Psychophysiology 2016;53(9):1366–76.

Adapting Well-Being into Outpatient Child Psychiatry

Sean Pustilnik, MD

KEYWORDS

- Mental health • Wellness • Well-being • Positive psychiatry
- Practice transformation • Child and adolescent • Measurement-based care
- Motivational interviewing

KEY POINTS

- Physical activity, nutrition, mindfulness, music, and arts are well-being interventions that can expand the focus of treatment toward enhancing mental health beyond patient and family symptoms and deficits.
- Measures addressing well-being are used during clinical assessment to clarify strengths and positive emotions that contribute to health.
- A collaborative, motivational interviewing approach can help patients and families adopt and track personalized well-being practices throughout treatment.

INTRODUCTION

Previous articles have described strategies to prioritize well-being, from evaluation and clinical assessment to inclusion of physical activity, music and arts, mindfulness, sleep, and nutrition to enhance treatment. The primary care setting is a natural site for well-being interventions. Primary care clinicians have substantial experience recommending exercise, good sleep, and nutrition in the course of treatment to improve physical illness and mental health difficulties. Child psychiatrists often address motivations and behaviors to help patients adopt healthier behaviors.

This article provides recommendations for incorporating well-being into an outpatient child and adolescent psychiatric practice, a setting traditionally focused more on symptoms and psychopathology. Outpatient practices can easily, gradually increase focus on building and fostering positive psychosocial characteristics, such as resilience, coping self-efficacy, social engagement, and optimism. Providers and practices may add well-being assessment and intervention incrementally to enhance

Disclosure Statement: None.
Division of Child and Adolescent Psychiatry, Medstar Georgetown University Hospital, Georgetown University School of Medicine, 2115 Wisconsin Avenue Northwest, Suite 200, Washington, DC 20007, USA
E-mail address: Sean.D.Pustilnik@gunet.georgetown.edu

Child Adolesc Psychiatric Clin N Am 28 (2019) 221–235
https://doi.org/10.1016/j.chc.2018.11.006
1056-4993/19/© 2018 Elsevier Inc. All rights reserved.

childpsych.theclinics.com

their assessment and treatments. The well-being approach represents a continuum as illustrated in **Table 1**.

OFFICE ENVIRONMENT AND PRECLINICAL ASSESSMENT

From the time of the initial telephone call or referral, office staff can obtain information about the reasons for seeking psychiatric care that include well-being. For instance, by eliciting goals for treatment, rather than just the presenting symptoms or difficulties, the practice can help facilitate engagement with the family and reduce stigma about seeking care. Practices may also update Web sites or marketing materials to reflect a well-being approach. For example, rather than listing typical mental illness conditions that are seen within the practice, describing treatments that promote positive mental health outcomes, such as life-satisfaction or self-acceptance, increase resilience, or promote recovery are increasingly common, such as http://www.mentalhealthamerica.net/every-child-needs and http://www.med.uvm.edu/vccyf/home.

The office can review aspects of the clinic's physical environment that promote well-being, such as positive signs promoting well-being and effective parenting within the office, pamphlets or magazines encouraging healthy nutrition and exercise for families, and bulletin boards promoting wellness activities (eg, local sports, music, art, theater opportunities). Postings of community resources and events that promote social engagement, mindfulness techniques, or groups also encourage well-being. Each

Table 1 Incremental approach toward adapting a well-being practice			
	Traditional Psychiatric Practice	**Approaching Well-Being Model**	**Robust Well-Being Model**
Targeted patients	Those with mental illness	Also at-risk populations	Add prevention and family members
Preclinic visit	Symptom checklists and rating scales	Add activities and strengths inventory	Description of positive psychosocial characteristics and environmental factors
Interview/ assessment	Focus on symptoms	Incorporate questions about well-being (eg, exercise, diet)	Assess resilience, optimism, self-efficacy, social engagement
Therapeutic focus	Symptom reduction, absence of criteria for mental illness	Improve diet and exercise, mindfulness	Increased well-being, satisfaction, life happiness
Use of medications	Target most impairing cluster of symptoms	In conjunction with other treatments, promote sleep	"Prescribe" 30-min physical activity, music, 10-min meditation
Follow-up assessment	Symptom rating scales and side-effect checks	Track health-promoting behaviors (sleep/diet)	Validated ratings of perceived stress vs coping self-efficacy
Office environment	Artwork and signage communicate tastes and needs of staff/ clinician	Diet and exercise magazines, pamphlets, community bulletins	Meditation/yoga room, embedded dietitian or health coach

Modified from Jeste DV, Palmer BW, Rettew DC, et al. Positive psychiatry: its time has come. J Clin Psychiatry 2015;76(6):676; with permission.

practice has unique staff interests around well-being, so implementing well-being practices within the office, such as daily morning meditation for staff or wellness walks at lunchtime, serve as powerful models promoting well-being, and embedding mental and physical health into patient care.

Preclinical assessments can be done by patients before (or at) their first visits, via scales that collect information and frame the assessment from a well-being perspective. Questions can be included to gage the patient's current well-being practices. In our own clinic, we start out by encouraging parents to list the child's strengths, hobbies, interests, and extracurricular activities at the beginning of the intake form. There are several questions about sleep habits, screen time, diet and nutrition, and relationships with peers and family interspersed between other traditional information, such as personal and family psychiatric history and presenting concerns and symptoms. **Box 1** shows well-being questions that can be added to intake forms.

Although it remains valuable to gather information about symptoms and diagnostic considerations to focus the clinical interview and assessment (eg, Vanderbilt Scales for attention-deficit/hyperactivity disorder [ADHD]), a shift to use of a broader questionnaire (eg, Behavior Assessment System for Children-3,)[1] enables clinicians to collect helpful information about symptoms and strengths. Scoring by staff before the initial clinical interview apprises the clinician of relevant symptom clusters, such

---

Box 1
Positive questions to add to the initial child psychiatry evaluation

Current Problem
  Child's strengths: Please describe what your child does well, such as sports, music, art, writing.
  How does your child cope with difficulties or frustrations?
  Child's hobbies (eg, building models, doing crafts, playing certain types of video games).
  Child's extracurricular activities: How did your child choose activities? Which ones will likely continue over the years?

Past Psychiatric History
  Has your child enjoyed counseling or talking to others about problems?
  Has your child implemented any mental health techniques learned from others?

Past Medical History
  Did your child have any medical issues to overcome/learn to do deal with?
  What does taking medicine mean to your child? Does your child adhere to medical treatments/plans?
  How did your child experience the birth of other siblings/adoptees (planned, eagerly anticipated, siblings/family member reactions?)
  How have your child's relationships progressed with other family members?

Developmental History
  Nutrition
    What are meal times like? How is your child's eating behavior and food choices?
  Sleep Behavior
    Does your child have a regular bedtime routine? What time does your child tend to get to sleep?
    How does sleep go (eg, enjoys, cuddles, stays in room, comes to sleep with others)?

Morning Routine
  How does your child get ready for school in the morning? Are there any enjoyable routines (eg, during breakfast, going to the bus, on the ride to school, picking out clothes)?

Education History
  How is your child's life at school? What does your child most enjoy at school? What classes/activities does your child most prefer?

as internalizing problems, hyperactivity, atypicality, or externalizing problems. This targets the psychiatric review of symptoms during the initial clinical encounter, leaving more time to focus on strengths, well-being practices, and a multifaceted plan that integrates diet, exercise, mindfulness, the arts, and the patient's interests and passions, beyond traditional medication management or deficit-focused psychotherapy. Other authors have described similar approaches of using a combination of informal questionnaires and broad-based standardized instruments, such as the Child Behavior Checklist[2] as in the Vermont Family Based Approach.[3] The Vermont Health and Behavior Questionnaire assesses additional domains of well-being, family structure and stability, self-esteem, family conflict and cohesion, and parenting practices. **Table 2** describes several of these broader screening instruments.

CLINICAL ASSESSMENT

Clinical assessment and interview components were detailed in this issue (See Schlechter, O'Brien, and Stewart: The Positive Assessment: Integrating Well-Being into the Clinical Evaluation, in this issue.) It is important for the clinician to structure the assessment sessions to elicit information from the child and family regarding strengths and assets beyond identified symptoms and deficiencies. As conceptualized by Keyes (**Fig. 1**), well-being is measured on its own dimensional axis from low to high, rather than describing mental illness symptoms as present or not.

Similar to symptoms in diabetes or other medical illness, clinicians may start with appropriate well-being behaviors, such as exercise or mindfulness, which impact living with a condition (whether diabetes or ADHD), and reduce the disease manifestations itself. For example, playing sports may be a valuable way for a child with ADHD to "use" motoric energy productively, or individual/small team sports may be an easier early step to sustain focus and to feel accomplishment. When performing the clinical assessment with children and families, the following four dimensions should be kept in mind[4]:

1. Deficiencies, symptoms, or underlying characteristics of the child
2. Risk factors in the environment or family
3. Strengths and assets of the child
4. Resources and opportunities in the environment or family for positive experiences

Although traditional clinical interview and mental state examination tends to focus primarily on dimension 1, with increasingly evaluations of dimensions 2, 3, and 4 further expand opportunities to enhance treatment. Most conditions typically billed require a designation within the first dimension. A systematic review of "the D's" (deficits, difficulties, disappointment, diagnoses, disease, disability, disempowerment, disenfranchisement, demoralization, dysfunction) requires identification of only atypical or aberrant qualities and may better clarify illness severity, but reinforces the illness identity[5] for children and by their parents. Lessons learned from the Strengths Model[6] and Person-Centered Care[7] models indicate that a focus on the child and family's goals and strengths is more productive than what the professional thinks is in their best interests or perceives they cannot do.

The following practices improve exploration of the well-being dimensions during the initial assessment:

- Allotting time to include PERMA-related questions (See Schlechter, O'Brien, and Stewart: The Positive Assessment: Integrating Well-Being into the Clinical Evaluation, in this issue.)

Table 2
Sample of broad-based measures with some assessment of well-being

Measure	Positive Domains	Versions	Ages (y)	Length/Time to Complete	Cost
Beck Youth Inventories	Self-concept inventory	Self-report	7–18	5 inventories of 20 questions, 5 min per inventory	Yes
Behavior Assessment System for Children	Adaptability, leadership, social skills and study skills	Teacher report Parent report Self-report	Preschool, 2–5 Child, 6–11 Adolescent, 12–21	100–185 items per scale (10–30 min depending on parent/teacher/self)	Yes
Behavioral and Emotional Rating Scale	Interpersonal/intrapersonal strength, family involvement, school functioning, affective strength, career strength	Teacher rating Parent rating Youth rating	5–18	52 items 10 min	Yes
Child Health Questionnaire	Physical functioning, general health perceptions, self-esteem, mental health, behavior	Parent report Child report	5–18 parent 10 + self	Self, 87 items Parent, 28 or 50 items	Free for research
Health of the National Outcome Scale for Children and Adolescents	Scholastic or language skills, emotional, peer relationships	Clinician Parent Self	Clinician/parent, 3–18 Self, 13–18	13 items 5 min	Free for UK services

(continued on next page)

Table 2
(continued)

Measure	Positive Domains	Versions	Ages (y)	Length/Time to Complete	Cost
Kidscreen	Physical/psychological well-being, moods/emotions, self-perception, autonomy, parent relations, social support, school environment, social acceptance, financial	Child report with parent proxy measure	8–18	10, 27, or 52 items	Free for research, manual purchase required
Strengths and Difficulties Questionnaire	Peer relationships and prosocial behavior along with impact supplement	Parent Teacher Self-report	Parent/teacher, 4–17 Self, 11–17	25 items 5 min	Free (paper version)
Youth Outcome Questionnaire	Interpersonal relations, critical items	Parent report and tracking Youth report and tracking	Parent, 4–17 Youth, 12–18	64 or 30 items	Yes

Adapted from Deighton J, Croudace T, Fonagy P, et al. Measuring mental health and wellbeing outcomes for children and adolescents to inform practice and policy: a review of child self-report measures. Child Adolesc Psychiatry Ment Health 2014;8:14; with permission.

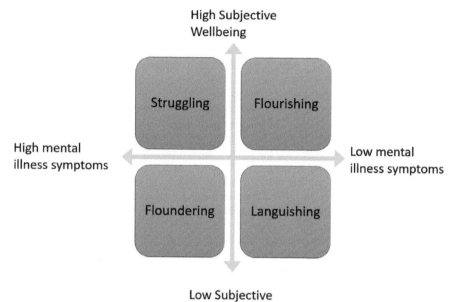

High Subjective
Wellbeing

Struggling   Flourishing

High mental   Low mental
illness symptoms   illness symptoms

Floundering   Languishing

Low Subjective
Wellbeing

Fig. 1. Dimensions of mental illness/health versus well-being. (*Adapted from* Keyes CLM, Lopez SJ. Toward a science of mental health: Positive directions in diagnosis and interventions. In: Snyder CR, Lopez SJ, editors. Handbook of Positive Psychology, Oxford University Press, New York, 2002:50.; with permission.)

- Breaking the evaluation into two sessions may be needed to capture symptoms and still allow identification of patient strengths/interests, and environmental supports/resources to optimize treatment.
- Reviewing screeners, scales, and demographic paperwork before the session allows less time to be allocated to symptom or deficit review (computer-based/scored instruments, or instruments easily scored by other staff may be preferable).
- Beginning the interview with child and family together, eliciting positive goals for treatment, and identifying the child (and family's) strengths and environmental factors "to work with."
- Wording may help families organize their input during the initial session: "I know that we are here today to talk about some things that have been difficult, so I'd like to get to those after we consider strengths we may be able to work with. (To child) What would you consider your strengths, or the things that you are best at? (To parents) How would you describe your child, what are his/her biggest strengths? (To both) What things do you do well together as a family?"
- Describing strengths about the child is disarming for parents (often expecting to quickly highlight the troubling symptoms), and leads to more open and balanced disclosure of deficits and adversities (ie, the parents see both the positive and negative sides of the situation rather than only the bleak).
- Conducting the assessment with child and parents present, or offering to save time at the end of the session, clarifies that any sensitive details from either party can be discussed safely.

PSYCHOEDUCATION: A DIMENSIONAL PERSPECTIVE

Once the clinician understands the patient's strengths and deficits, the clinician can provide impressions of shared concerns, and map out treatment. In traditional models, this process often relies on the disease or illness perspective, explaining symptoms by biochemical, neuroanatomic, or psychopathologic underpinnings, frustrating families when symptoms do not fit categorical description. An alternative psychoeducation approach is the dimensional perspective,[8] where human characteristics that are present and adaptive in the general population may become overexpressesd or underexpressed and become less adaptive or problematic. A simple example to help families understand is "height." We know what an average height is, and what measurements constitute short versus tall. One would not say that tall or short is a disorder; however, as shown in **Fig. 2**, when the very tall person buys a bed or a car, or flies in a plane, such situations create difficulty and may lead to dysfunction (eg, resistance to flying, concluding one is not "okay" because the world is not designed for the person to fit in).

Similarly, for a condition like ADHD,[9] parents can be educated in terms of a dimensional ability to sustain attention. At one end of the spectrum are people who are able to sustain focus on one task for a long period of time, perhaps appearing even obsessive or rigid. On the other end are those with more high energy, novelty seeking, craving of multiple simultaneous sensory inputs, or who prefer jumping from one topic to the next quickly. From an evolutionary standpoint, this may have been adaptive in terms of being able to shift attention quickly to recognize danger approaching or scout for food stores. However, with the pressing demands to sustain attention for educational environments and the ever-intruding stimuli of our electronic society, this phenotype may create dysfunction in today's school and family environments. In this way,

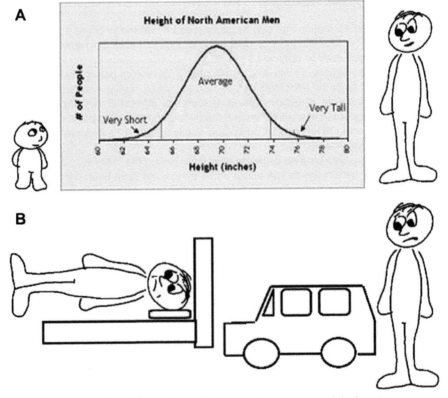

Fig. 2. (*A, B*) Dimensional illustrations of height leading to sense of dysfunction.

such medications as stimulants need not be viewed as restoring some pathologic brain dysfunction as in the disease model, but rather as promoting an inherent ability to sustain attention that is less expressed in this individual patient, as shown in **Fig. 3**.

Another example is anxiety (**Fig. 4**), where evidence supports a dimensional classification.[10] Most parents accept that every person has some degree of anxiety, and having some anxiety is useful. If a child had no anxiety at all, he or she might not go to school or do their homework, because of too little worry or concern about failing their classes or being ready for the future. At some point, however, anxiety becomes counterproductive once the person experiences too much, becoming paralyzed by fearing failure, or having preoccupations preventing concentration on the task at hand. Treatment is conceptualized as reducing excess anxiety back to an optimal level for productiveness, either with psychotherapeutic techniques, medication, or a combination. A simplified version of this is to have the child point to where on the graph (**Figs. 4** and **5**) they believe represents their current level of anxiety and functioning.

A dimensional approach helps for many other conditions, even when an illness-based or categorical approach may be easier for a family to accept ("oh, that's because of ADHD, not laziness"). By explaining presenting symptoms as an overexpression or underexpression of traits that lie on a continuum with typical, this normalizes the experience for the patient and family, decreasing stigma, and provides an entry point to discuss and measure treatment interventions.

USE OF MEDICATIONS AND NONPHARMACOLOGIC PRESCRIPTIONS

The discussion of medication use is focused more toward promoting a sense of well-being and positive emotions with the PERMA approach.[11] **Table 3** provides questions to integrate PERMA into medication evaluation and treatment.

The discussion of medication can also focus on promotion of health goals, such as sleep-inducing medications being viewed to enhance restorative sleep, rather than to treat insomnia. Stimulants may be discussed as promoting ability to sustain attention instead of reducing poor focus or hyperactivity. Selective serotonin reuptake inhibitors (SSRIs) could be considered promoting a sense of calm or happiness instead of reducing anxiety and depression. Even mood stabilizers or antipsychotics, if necessary, can be considered as promoting reality testing and for maintaining a steady

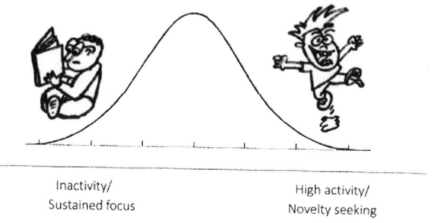

Inactivity/
Sustained focus

High activity/
Novelty seeking

Fig. 3. Dimensional representation of ADHD.

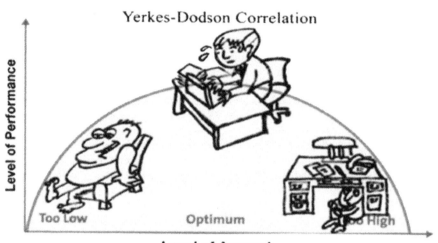

Fig. 4. Dimensional representation of anxiety. (*Adapted from* Yerkes RM, Dodson JD. The relation of strength of stimulus to rapidity of habit-formation. J Comp Neurology Psychol 1908;18(5):479; with permission.)

mood. Defining improvement toward desired goals (eg, "How much will you sleep?" "How long will you be able to sustain attention?" "What will calmness look and feel like if the SSRI is effective?" "What will happen to your grandiose thoughts if treatment works?") can replace the deficit, symptom-focused model, where health is described as the absence of undesirable symptoms (eg, "Are you still waking up every night?" "Are you still having trouble finishing school tasks?" "How sad/suicidal are you today?" "Are you still having mood fluctuations daily?"). In this latter encounter, patients may feel known as having "undesirable" attributes rather than recognized for their positive ones; even implicitly, attention is provided patients around distressing

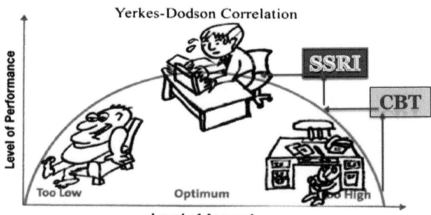

Fig. 5. Treatment effects on a dimensional model of anxiety. CBT, cognitive behavioral therapy; SSRI, selective serotonin reuptake inhibitor. (*Adapted from* Yerkes RM, Dodson JD. The relation of strength of stimulus to rapidity of habit-formation. J Comp Neurology Psychol 1908;18(5):479; with permission.)

Table 3	
Well-being-based psychopharmacology evaluation	
Positive emotions	What positive emotions do you hope to regain or feel more (if you take a medication)? What would you wish treatment could alter about your current emotions? How do you currently feel: Serenity? Hope? Awe? Love? Joy? Inspiration? Gratitude?
Engagement	How able are you to engage in the things that matter most to you? What activities do you lose yourself in? What are you now noticing about losing yourself in those activities?
Relationships	How are you connecting to others currently? How will those close to you think about your diagnosis? How would they react to you taking medications?
Meaning	What things have meaning to you? How do you spend most of your time? What does it mean to have a psychiatric diagnosis? To take a medication?
Accomplishment	What are you accomplishing these days, or continuing to do well? What is getting in the way of you being able to do what you want to? What do you hope treatment helps you to accomplish?

Courtesy of J. Bostic, MD, EdD, Washington, DC.

symptoms, so treatment encounters may seem focused on remaining sick for the patient to sustain interaction with the treater.

Most of the research behind pharmacotherapy centers around concepts of response (drop in symptom severity) or even (optimistically) remission (absence of symptoms sufficient to meet criteria for disease). Medication interventions alone is likely insufficient for remission or for achieving well-being for individual patients.[12] Rather, other interventions are necessary in combination with pharmacotherapy. This serves to bridge families who are reticent to considering psychotropic medications and to help families explore multimodal aspects of a treatment plan focused on well-being interventions.

Just as informing a family of the relative efficacy of an SSRI medication for treatment of depression, the clinician can describe the relative strength and efficacy of well-being-based interventions. Explaining that physical activity can have positive effects on symptoms of depression[13] and ADHD,[14] healthy diet can reduce incidence of externalizing behavior disorders,[15] and that meditation can have positive effects on physical and mental health outcomes in kids[16] can lend credence to the psychiatrist practicing evidence-based medicine and promoting well-being. "Prescribing" these practices, by actually writing several on a prescription (**Fig. 6**), provides a powerful message to patients and families about altering patterns around health-promoting behaviors.[17]

Selecting several, viable, appealing healthy interventions can be measured and tracked (ie, not all of the possible healthy practices should be prescribed at once). Interventions can be supplemented with appropriate patient and family instruction on these interventions. For example, if the family seems interested and motivated to improve healthy eating habits, they are directed to such sites as https://www.choosemyplate.gov/myplate-tip-sheets. Many families prefer electronic or app-based information and tracking, such as available at www.calorieking.com or the MyFitnessPal app. Based on family preferences, similar print or electronic information is given related to exercise, meditation and relaxation interventions, music and art activities, social engagement strategies, and positive parenting practices.

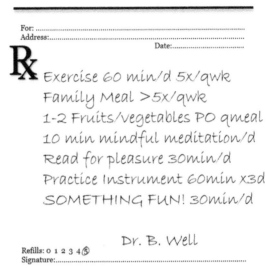

For: ....
Address:...
                                Date:...............................

R̶x̶ Exercise 60 min/d 5x/qwk
Family Meal >5x/qwk
1-2 Fruits/vegetables PO qmeal
10 min mindful meditation/d
Read for pleasure 30min/d
Practice Instrument 60min x3d
SOMETHING FUN! 30min/d

Dr. B. Well

Refills: 0 1 2 3 4 ⑤
Signature:...

Fig. 6. Prescription for several well-being interventions.

FOLLOW-UP MEETINGS AND INTERVENTIONS

Subsequent meetings allow the clinician to track improvement of symptoms, and to assess well-being behavior progress and attempts toward positive emotional experiences. Some clinicians start each session with a 5- to 10-minute mindfulness practice or other relaxation strategy, such as deep abdominal breathing, progressive muscle relaxation, guided imagery, or yoga poses. This can help to put the child and family in a relaxed state of mind and ready to work during the session. These practices can also be reinforced by assigning home-based relaxation practice, using appropriate search terms for the youth or family member to type into a search engine or You-Tube (eg, "guided meditation for kids").

Follow-up rating scales, or individualized measurement using more informal scaling questions, are reviewed to track progress, including follow-up PERMA assessments:

- How has your mood been since our last meeting on a scale from 1 to 10?
- What emotions have you experienced the most often, or most intensely? Rate them 1 to 10.
- How are you engaging? How are relationships going with others? What are you accomplishing?
- What has it meant to you to be taking medications?

Families can measure outcomes related to wellness goals by tracking the amount of time spent on each activity per day, such as with a standard Task Planning and Achievement Log found in standard cognitive behavioral therapy approaches **(Table 4)**. It is important to be specific and measurable when negotiating homework, and setting realistic, attainable goals.

Some families and providers prefer technology-based tracking, such as wearable devices to monitor physical activity, exercise levels, sleep quality, and dietary logs and calorie counters. Use of meditation apps also provides data to the user and clinician regarding frequency of use. Apps can also be used to track mood ratings multiple

Table 4
Example of a standard task planning and achievement log

Task or Activity	Monday	Tuesday	Wednesday	Thursday	Friday	Saturday	Sunday
Deep breathing practice, 5 times/day	✓✓✓✓✓	✓✓✓✓✓	✓✓✓	✓✓✓✓✓✓✓	✓✓✓✓✓	✓✓✓✓	✓✓
Eat breakfast	✓	✓		✓		✓	✓
Play tennis 30 min, 4 times this wk	30 min		20 min	45 min		60 min	
Sleep 8–9 h	8 h	7 h	9 h	6 h	8 h	10 h	9 h

times daily rather than paper mood logs or journals. Apps listed next cross several categories that may appeal to various patients:

- Mood tracking: Dailyo, Mood Panda, iMood, Happier, In Flow, Moodtrack Diary, Emotionary
- Meditation: Calm, Headspace, Stop Breathe & Think, Smiling Mind, Insight Timer, Grow, Zazen, 7-s Meditation, Breathe2Relax, 10% Happier
  - Palousemindfulness.com also offers a free full online course on mindful meditation
- Nutrition: Fat Secret, Calorie King, MyFitnesspal, MyPlate, Meal Snap, Fooducate, Healthy Heroes, Eat and Move-o-Matic, Perfect Picnic
- Fitness: C-Fit Yoga, DownDog, Super Stretch Yoga HD, Fitness Kids, Iron Kids, FitQuest Lite
- Wearable devices with apps: Vivofit Jr, Fitbit Ace, Kidfit, Leapfrog, Vtech Kidizoom, Nabi, Sqord

Because almost all of the well-being interventions described are related to behavioral change, a motivational interviewing approach is helpful to clarify goals for the child and family and review any barriers to implementation. Simple interventions are usually easier at first. The sample questions listed next can help facilitate the goal-setting process with well-being-based interventions:

- Can you tell me how exercising more might benefit your health, or how you have been feeling?
- How important do you think it would be to exercise more, on a scale from 1 to 10?
- What makes it a 7 (whatever number patient said), and not say a 1 or 2? What makes it a 7 and not a 9 or 10?
- What would be a realistic goal to set for the number of times you will exercise this week? And for how much time should we shoot for? What type of activities do you think you will do?
- How realistic do you think it will be to exercise four times this week for 30 minutes? On a scale from 1 to 10?
- What makes it a 6 and not a 3? What makes it a 6 and not a 10? How could we get it to 10?
- Identify any potential barriers and brainstorm solutions together.

Other types of psychotherapeutic interventions fostering positive emotions can be delivered during the session, with the patient or family included.

- Using Strengths: List five strengths that best describe you. Brainstorm how to use them more this week.

- 3 Good Things: Journal nightly of three specific good things that happened that day.
- Gratitude Letter: Write a letter to someone you are grateful for but never thanked. Read it to them.
- Savoring: Slowly enjoy something for 2 to 3 minutes with all five senses at least twice per day.

Families are encouraged to do these tasks together, such as listing three good things during their evening meal (or if this is difficult "rose, thorn, bud"—one good, one difficult, and one to look forward to). A focus on positive parenting including reinforcers and attention for positive behaviors can also be helpful for families implementing a well-being approach.

BUILDING A TEAM

Whether in a solo or large practice group, everything discussed in this article can be suitably adapted, including helping practices better use a team approach. The psychiatrist might model working with others and demonstrate healthy relationships by teaming up and collaborate toward patient's well-being. Other mental health clinicians might then act in the role of health coach or family coach responsible for organizing and tracking well-being interventions, such as exercise, nutrition, mindfulness, and arts. They may focus more on at-risk families, whereas a psychologist provides family psychotherapy to more symptomatic families.

Different providers can dedicate efforts to specific well-being practices, and this may help achieve a comprehensive plan (ie, a therapist in the office who has interest in mindfulness or yoga could lead group meditation or exercise classes). Group interventions may be particularly effective ways to deliver positive coping interventions and have participants practice these with input from nonclinician peers. Clinicians may choose to partner with other community professionals who can promote these interventions who offer nutrition support, health coaching or personal training to promote physical activity, music performance, or artistic efforts.

SUMMARY

Practical guidance is emerging for implementing a continuum of well-being into the child psychiatry outpatient clinic. Starting with the initial encounter, psychoeducation, exploring medication options, and well-being interventions can be implemented with motivational interviewing approaches. Tracking and monitoring progress during follow-up, integrating electronic resources, and adding positive psychotherapeutic techniques even with medication interventions all incorporate well-being into all facets of treatment. This positions the child psychiatrist to shift from focus on symptoms and deficit mental illness toward positive psychosocial characteristics to help children thrive.

REFERENCES

1. Sandoval J, Echandia A. Behavior assessment system for children. J Sch Psychol 1994;32:419–25.
2. Achenbach TM, Rescorla LA. TMRLA: manual for the ASEBA school-age forms and profiles. Burlington (NJ): University of Vermont Research Center for Children, Youth, and Families; 2001.
3. Hudziak JJ. Genetic and environmental influences on wellness, resilience, and psychopathology: a family based approach for promotion, prevention, and

intervention. In: Hudziak JJ, editor. Developmental psychopathology and wellness: genetic and environmental influences. Washington, DC: American Psychiatric Publishing; 2008. p. 267–86.

4. Wright BA, Lopez SJ. Widening the diagnostic focus. A case for including human strengths and environmental resources. In: Snyder CR, Lopez SJ, editors. Handbook of positive psychology. New York: Oxford University Press; 2002. p. 26–44.
5. Slade M. Mental illness and well-being: the central importance of positive psychology and recovery approaches. BMC Health Serv Res 2010;10:26.
6. Rapp C, Goscha RJ. The strengths model: case management with people with psychiatric disabilities, vol. 2. New York: Oxford University Press; 2006.
7. Tondora J, Pocklington S, Osher D, et al. Implementation of person-centered care and planning: from policy to practice to evaluation. Washington, DC: Substance Abuse and Mental Health Services Administration; 2005.
8. Helzer JE, Kraemer HC, Krueger RF. The feasibility and need for dimensional psychiatric diagnoses. Psychol Med 2006;36:1671–80.
9. Marcus DK, Barry TD. Does attention-deficit/hyperactivity disorder have a dimensional latent structure? A taxometric analysis. J Abnorm Psychol 2011;120(2): 427–42.
10. Beesdo K, Knappe S, Pine DS. Anxiety and anxiety disorders in children and adolescents: developmental issues and implications for DSM-V. Psychiatr Clin North Am 2009;32(3):483–524.
11. Seligman MEP. Flourish: a visionary new understanding of happiness and well-being. New York: Free Press; 2011.
12. Rettew D. Positive child psychiatry [Chapter 14]. In: Jeste DV, Palmer BW, editors. Positive psychiatry: a clinical handbook. Arlington, VA: American Psychiatric Publishing; 2015. p. 285–304.
13. Carter T, Morres ID, Meade O, et al. The effect of exercise on depressive symptoms in adolescents: a systematic review and meta-analysis. J Am Acad Child Adolesc Psychiatry 2016;55:580–90.
14. Smith AL, Hoza B, Linnea K, et al. Pilot physical activity intervention reduces severity of ADHD symptoms in young children. J Atten Disord 2013;17(1):70–82.
15. Jacka FN, Ystrom E, Brantsaeter AL, et al. Maternal and early postnatal nutrition and mental health of offspring by age 5 years: a prospective cohort study. J Am Acad Child Adolesc Psychiatry 2013;52(10):1038–47.
16. Black DS, Milam J, Sussman S. Sitting-meditation interventions among youth: a review of treatment efficacy. Pediatrics 2009;124(3):e532–41.
17. Hudziak J. Child psychiatry: this is where we build healthy brains. Oral presentation at the 64th annual meeting of the American Academy of Child & Adolescent Psychiatry in Washington DC, October 27, 2017.

Emerging Topics in Well-Being

Health Promotion in Primary Care Pediatrics

Initial Results of a Randomized Clinical Trial of the Vermont Family Based Approach

Masha Y. Ivanova, PhD[a],*, Lauren Dewey, PhD[a],
Pamela Swift, PhD[a], Stanley Weinberger, MD[b], Jim Hudziak, MD[a,c]

KEYWORDS

- Vermont Family Based Approach • Family wellness coaching
- Healthcare innovation • Randomized controlled (clinical) trial
- Mental health in pediatrics • Integrated care

KEY POINTS

- The Vermont Family Based Approach (VFBA) is an innovative approach to healthcare delivery that addresses many significant challenges of the current healthcare system in the United States.
- A randomized controlled trial (RCT) of the VFBA was conducted at a primary care pediatric clinic.
- The RCT aimed to test the feasibility of the VFBA in primary care pediatrics and to improve healthcare engagement and health outcomes for children and parents.
- This article presents the initial results of the trial on feasibility and engagement.
- The VFBA was feasible in primary care pediatrics and was associated with a significant increase in engagement with health and wellness supports and services for families.

INTRODUCTION

The healthcare delivery system in the United States (US) is facing significant challenges.[1,2] Novel, effective approaches to the delivery of healthcare that address the endemic problems of the current system are needed. The Vermont Family Based Approach (VFBA) is an innovative approach to healthcare delivery that aims to overcome several serious challenges affecting the US healthcare system.[3,4]

Disclosure Statement: None to disclose.
[a] Department of Psychiatry, University of Vermont, 1 South Prospect Street, Burlington, VT 05401, USA; [b] Department of Pediatrics, University of Vermont, 1 South Prospect Street, Burlington, VT 05401, USA; [c] Medicine, Pediatrics and Communication Sciences and Disorders, University of Vermont, 1 South Prospect Street, Burlington, VT 05401, USA
* Corresponding author.
E-mail address: Masha.Ivanova@uvm.edu

Child Adolesc Psychiatric Clin N Am 28 (2019) 237–246
https://doi.org/10.1016/j.chc.2018.11.005
1056-4993/19/© 2018 Elsevier Inc. All rights reserved.

childpsych.theclinics.com

The Vermont Family Based Approach

The VFBA is a population-based approach to healthcare delivery.[3] The VFBA organizes healthcare around the entire family rather than the individual. The family is viewed as the primary health promoting social institution that disseminates health-related attitudes, beliefs, and practices.[5,6] The VFBA also brings emotional and behavioral health to the center of healthcare. Emotional and behavioral problems predict or influence the course of all major nonpsychiatric medical conditions.[7] They are also the most costly health conditions in the US.[8] To make significant improvements in population health, we need approaches to healthcare delivery that directly address emotional and behavioral health. Another important feature of the VFBA is that it emphasizes health promotion and prevention of illness. This feature is based on overwhelming empirical evidence that health promotion and prevention are powerful determinants of health across the life span.[9]

Family Wellness Coaching

The VFBA is a team-based approach that brings together health and wellness professionals to partner with families. As part of each family's team, the VFBA introduces a new healthcare professional, the Family Wellness Coach. The Family Wellness Coach is a bachelor's degree–level or master's degree–level health professional who has received training in family wellness coaching. The Family Wellness Coach works with families on a comprehensive program of health and wellness that is individualized to each family. The program addresses the evidence-based wellness domains of nutrition, exercise, mindfulness, sleep, positive parenting, creative arts, and community involvement.[1]

The Family Wellness Coach directly coaches family members in these wellness domains and connects them to community partners specializing in specific aspects of health promotion (eg, certified swimming instructors or music educators), where appropriate. In addition to helping families develop and implement their individualized wellness programs, the Family Wellness Coach also serves as a liaison between the family and the rest of the family's healthcare team. When needed, the Family Wellness Coach also helps families to address problems of living, such as transportation, housing, and food insecurity. Families meet with their Family Wellness Coaches in the clinic or community.

Because the VFBA strongly emphasizes emotional and behavioral health, one important responsibility of the Family Wellness Coach is to assess and continuously monitor the emotional and behavioral health of family members using empirically based assessment instruments. If results of assessment indicate that a family member is experiencing significant emotional and behavioral problems, the Family Wellness Coach connects them with Focused Family Coaches and Family-Based Psychiatrists. Focused Family Coaches are credentialed psychotherapists who offer treatment from the family perspective. This includes individual treatment of both child and adult family members and family-based psychotherapy. Family-Based Psychiatrists provide psychiatric care from the family perspective also by treating both child and adult family members. An important aspect of the VFBA is that Family Wellness Coaches, Focused Family Coaches, and Family-Based Psychiatrists all use evidence-based approaches for health promotion and treatment.

Advantages of the Vermont Family Based Approach

The VFBA addresses several serious challenges affecting the US healthcare delivery system. First, organizing the delivery of healthcare services around the family system rather than around individuals reduces the redundancy and increases the coordination of care. Second, because Family Wellness Coaches are in frequent contact with families and because other members of the VFBA healthcare team actively practice health promotion and prevention as part of their professional scope of practice, the entire healthcare delivery system shifts its emphasis from illness and disease to health promotion and prevention. Third, Family Wellness Coaches help family members to monitor the emotional and behavioral health of all family members and connect family members to Focused Family Coaches and Family-Based Psychiatrists, as soon as there is need for mental health services. In so doing, they facilitate timely access to professional emotional and behavioral care, preventing problems from getting entrenched. Finally, because Family Wellness Coaches are trained in basic evidence-based interventional approaches, they may help families ameliorate mild emotional and behavioral problems and parenting difficulties, eliminating the need for referral to Focused Family Coaches and Family-Based Psychiatrists. This may help enhance the capacity of the healthcare system and reduce clinician burden.

The Pilot Randomized Clinical Trial of the Vermont Family Based Approach in a Primary Care Pediatric Clinic

In this article, the authors describe a recently completed first randomized clinical (controlled) trial (RCT) of the VFBA and present its initial findings on feasibility and healthcare engagement. The RCT tested the feasibility and efficacy of the VFBA in the University of Vermont Children's Hospital Pediatric Primary Care Clinic (UVM Pediatrics). The RCT was sponsored by the University of Vermont Medical Center (UVM MC). Although the interventional elements comprising the VFBA have been supported by empirical evidence, the whole approach has not yet been rigorously tested in the RCT framework.

UVM Pediatrics is a community-based primary care pediatric clinic that serves Burlington, Vermont, and surrounding communities. Burlington is the largest city in Vermont, with a population of over 42,000 residents living in more than 16,000 households.[10] The population of Burlington is primarily White/non-Hispanic (84%), with Asian (6%), Black/African American (4.9%), and Hispanic/Latino (2.6%) residents comprising the largest minority communities. The median household income is approximately $47,000, and approximately 25% of Burlington's residents live below the federal poverty level.[10]

We chose to conduct the first RCT of the VFBA at UVM Pediatrics believing that ideas of family-based care and health promotion would resonate with primary care pediatricians, who deal with both parents and children and strongly emphasize health promotion in their work with families.

Goals of the Randomized Clinical Trial and of this Article

The RCT of the VFBA at UVM Pediatrics was conducted primarily to test the feasibility of the VFBA in a community primary care pediatric clinic. As a secondary goal, the RCT aimed to test the efficacy of the VFBA to improve healthcare engagement and health outcomes for children and parents. This article presents the initial feasibility and engagement results of the RCT and aims to answer the following questions:

1. Is the VFBA model feasible in a real-life, primary care pediatric setting?
2. Do families engage with Family Wellness Coaches?
3. Is the VFBA associated with a significant increase in engagement with health and wellness supports and services?

METHOD
Pre-Planning

Before commencing the study, the research team met regularly with the UVM Pediatrics practitioners and support staff for 4 months to ensure that the developing study procedures were ecologically sound and acceptable to them. All aspects of the protocol were designed with their input.

Design

The study used an RCT design with open randomization. Using rolling recruitment, we recruited families to the RCT from December 2015 to December, 2017. We also recruited nine additional families to the VFBA group to increase our power to better characterize the VFBA. However, the data for the nine non-randomized families are not presented in this paper.

The data for the 9 nonrandomized families, however, are not presented in this article. For randomized families, data collection concluded in June 2018, to allow families who were recruited in December 2017 to receive at least 6 months of the intervention. The dose of the received intervention thus ranged from 6 months to 30 months.

Eligibility Criteria

The study was originally designed for families with 3 year olds to 6 year olds, whose children were presenting for routine primary care at UVM Pediatrics. Parents were required to be proficient enough in English to complete the assessment materials, and at least 1 parent needed to consent to study participation from the family. The RCT was originally planned as a 12-month feasibility and instrumentation pilot. Because the UVM MC extended its funding of the project beyond the 12-month period, we expanded the upper age of the target children to 15 years during the second year of recruitment to broaden our understanding of the effects of the VFBA across children's development.

Sample Characteristics

Participants were 81 children and families who were randomized to the VFBA or control groups. The child sample was 46% female (37 girls and 44 boys) and primarily of preschool age at baseline assessment (Mean = 4.89; SD = 1.88; range: 3–14 years old).

The majority of children were White, non-Hispanic (53 [65%]). The remaining group was diverse: 10 children were of African descent (12%); 3 (3.7%) of Asian, Hispanic, and Nepali descent each; 5 of Middle Eastern descent (6%); and 4 (5%) of mixed descent. The sample was more racially and ethnically diverse than the Burlington community, as described previously.

To describe the socioeconomic status (SES) of the sample, we used the Hollingshead SES index for parental occupations updated by Achenbach.[11,12] Based on parental occupations, a numeric SES score was assigned, ranging from 10 (low SES) to 90 (high SES), to each family. In 2-parent households, the higher score was selected. SES scores ranged from 10 to 90 (Mean = 53.95; SD = 25.92; 25th percentile = 30; 50th percentile = 50; and 75th percentile = 80). For 21 families (26%), the SES score was at or below 30, indicating the very low to low range (ie, unemployed, unskilled, or semiskilled worker). The sample was thus diverse with respect to SES.

Procedures

All study procedures were approved by the UVM Institutional Review Board. Eligible families were identified weekly by screening upcoming routine clinic appointments.

Visual reminders about a family's eligibility for the study were placed in the children's visit folders to prompt pediatric practitioners to introduce the study to families. After the appointment, research staff contacted interested families and consented them in person at their preferred location. After completing a comprehensive baseline assessment, families were randomized to the VFBA or control groups. All families completed interim assessments every 4 months to 6 months and a final comprehensive assessment.

The VFBA group received ongoing family wellness coaching, therapeutic assessment feedback, and a partnership with a Focused Family Coach and/or a family-based psychiatrist, if indicated by results of their baseline assessment. The Focused Family Coaches and Family-Based Psychiatrists were available to see them immediately. The VFBA group also received a menu of optional, cost-free wellness offerings, including violin instruction for children and parents, parenting classes, swimming lessons, and family events (with childcare and dinner provided) that focused mostly on mindfulness and nutrition. Music recitals for violin students were held twice a year and were followed by dinner celebrations.

The VFBA team met weekly for care planning and coordination, and the Family Wellness Coaches communicated regularly with the children's pediatrics practitioners. We used an online care coordination platform, ACT.md to facilitate communication between the VFBA team, pediatric practitioners, and families. Families in the VFBA group were not remunerated for participation.

The control group received care as usual at UVM Pediatrics. They were also remunerated for completing study assessments (ie, $100 for the comprehensive baseline and final assessments plus $50 for each smaller interim assessment).

Assessment Instruments

As part of larger assessments, parents completed the Health Supports and Services Questionnaire (HSSQ), which was designed for this study. The HSSQ asks respondents whether members of their family have looked into or received health and wellness supports and services aimed at emotional and behavioral health and wellness. Respondents are asked about both looking into and receiving the supports and services to assess both the precontemplative and action stages of behavior change. Families in both groups completed the HSSQ at baseline, final, and interim assessments as a paper-and-pencil questionnaire. After each contact with families, Family Wellness Coaches completed the Family Contact Questionnaire, which was also developed for this project. The Family Contact Questionnaire describes the Family Wellness Coach's contact with the family, including who initiated the contact and the contact's topic and modality (ie, in-person, phone, text message, e-mail, or video-conferencing). The Family Wellness Coaches completed the contact in ACT.md electronically after each contact with families.

RESULTS
Question 1: Is the Vermont Family Based Approach Model Feasible in a Real-Life, Primary Care Pediatric Setting?

Pediatric primary care is a high-paced and hectic environment. Our successful implementation of study procedures and participant recruitment at UVM Pediatrics indicated that the VFBA was feasible in this environment. Furthermore, per the UVM MC policy, only treating clinicians are allowed to introduce interventional research opportunities to the UVM MC patients, and researchers are prohibited from doing so. Because of this policy, recruitment was entirely in the hands of the pediatric practitioners. Their referral of patients to the authors' study indicated that they saw value in the VFBA.

Question 2: Did Families Engage with Family Wellness Coaches?

Because the Family Wellness Coach is a new kind of healthcare professional, it was important to test whether families would engage with Family Wellness Coaches. Using the Family Contact Questionnaire, Family Wellness Coaches reported 1672 contacts with families over the course of the study. These ranged from 3 to 120 per family (mean = 36.35; SD = 25.51; 25th percentile = 17.75; 50th percentile = 27.50; and 75th percentile = 47.25). At 545 (33%) and 531 (32%) contacts, in-person and e-mail contacts were the most frequent communication modalities, followed by text messages (334/20%), phone calls (253/15%), videoconferences (4/0.2%), or unknown (5/0.3%)) types of contacts.

   Fig. 1 presents frequencies of topics that were addressed during the Family Wellness Coaches' contacts with families. They add up to greater than 1672 because more than 1 topic could have been addressed during a contact. The 3 most frequent topics addressed during contacts were exercise (640/23%), mindfulness (473/17%), and child emotional and behavioral care (418/15%).

Question 3: Was the Vermont Family Based Approach Associated with a Significant Increase in Engagement with Health and Wellness Supports and Services?

We used general linear modeling repeated measures analyses to compare rates of change in engagement with health and wellness supports and services for the VFBA and control groups. We specified a full factorial model with all factors and inter-actions and without covariates. Engagement with health and wellness supports and services was measured by the HSSQ scores listed in **Table 1**.

   To define the within-subject factor of engagement with health and wellness sup-ports and services, we compared mean HSSQ scores obtained at baseline vs. over the course of the study. The latter was calculated as a sum of HSSQ scores obtained at all assessment periods since baseline available for a family. The number of HSSQ scores that were obtained since baseline varied across families because rolling recruitment was used.

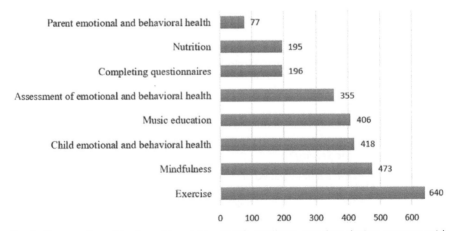

Fig. 1. Frequencies of topics addressed by Family Wellness Coaches during contacts with families.

Table 1
Descriptive statistics for number of health and wellness supports and services looked into or received at baseline and over the course of the study (during study) by group

Type of Health Supports and Services	Vermont Family Based Approach		Control		P Time × Group Interaction
	Baseline Mean (SD)	During Study Mean (SD)	Baseline Mean (SD)	During Study Mean (SD)	
Looked into					
1. Exercise and fitness training	1.12 (1.32)	6.15 (4.81)	1.07 (1.33)	2.63 (3.13)	.002
2. Nutrition training	0.36 (0.82)	1.94 (2.61)	0.50 (0.91)	1.46 (2.06)	.316
3. Mindfulness training	0.47 (0.99)	3.62 (3.63)	0.73 (1.08)	1.00 (2.12)	<.0001
4. Music training	0.36 (0.65)	4.67 (3.70)	0.38 (0.85)	1.12 (1.53)	<.0001
5. Sleep-related services	0.12 (0.41)	1.09 (1.85)	0.44 (1.04)	0.56 (1.23)	.053
6. Vocational services	0.26 (0.56)	0.33 (0.92)	0.30 (0.72)	0.26 (0.71)	.660
7. Support group	0.35 (0.81)	1.56 (2.48)	0.40 (0.91)	0.60 (1.32)	.069
8. Psychotherapy	0.74 (1.05)	3.74 (3.61)	0.96 (0.84)	1.16 (1.75)	<.0001
9. Psychiatric care	0.34 (0.70)	1.34 (1.98)	0.48 (0.92)	1.16 (1.77)	.500
10. Substance-related care	0.03 (0.18)	0.16 (0.58)	0.13 (0.61)	0.00 (0.00)	.116
12. Support regarding problems of living	0.29 (0.46)	0.79 (0.99)	0.30 (0.47)	0.48 (0.79)	.134
Received					
1. Exercise and fitness training	0.96 (1.14)	5.44 (4.27)	0.73 (0.94)	2.18 (2.40)	.003
2. Nutrition training	0.48 (0.95)	2.35 (4.11)	0.25 (0.55)	1.05 (1.43)	.207
3. Mindfulness training	0.60 (1.19)	4.25 (4.20)	0.39 (0.61)	0.83 (1.47)	.004
4. Music training	0.14 (0.36)	4.81 (4.06)	0.11 (0.32)	0.61 (0.92)	<.0001
5. Sleep-related services	0.11 (0.46)	0.53 (1.61)	0.22 (0.55)	0.50 (1.15)	.718
6. Vocational services	0.18 (0.39)	0.18 (0.50)	0.18 (0.53)	0.24 (0.75)	.621
7. Support group	0.20 (0.62)	0.85 (1.46)	0.32 (0.48)	0.95 (1.61)	.972
8. Psychotherapy	0.56 (0.77)	3.16 (2.67)	0.67 (0.70)	1.17 (1.43)	.001
9. Psychiatric care	0.42 (0.84)	1.16 (2.09)	0.18 (0.39)	1.29 (1.83)	.574
10. Substance-related care	0.19 (0.54)	0.12 (0.34)	0.59 (0.24)	0.18 (0.73)	.337
11. Support regarding problems of living	0.30 (0.46)	0.80 (1.04)	0.25 (0.44)	0.65 (0.99)	.709

P = P of the interaction of time of assessment (baseline vs over the course of the study) and group (VFBA vs control).

Over the course of the study, being in the VFBA group was associated with a significantly steeper increase in both looking into and receiving exercise and fitness, mindfulness and music training, and psychotherapy in comparison to the control group (see **Table 1**). For looking into sleep services and support groups, the difference favoring the VFBA group approached statistical significance. The last column of **Table 1** lists the P values for the interaction terms of group (VFBA vs control) and time of assessment (baseline vs over the course of the study), which compare the rate of change between the 2 groups. To illustrate these interactions, we plotted the interaction for the first effect presented in **Table 1** (looked into exercise and fitness) in **Fig. 2**. The plots for other significant interactions were similar.

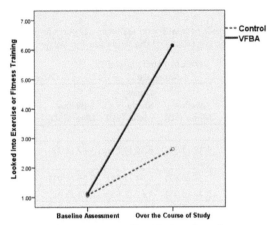

Fig. 2. Interaction of group (VFBA vs control) with time (baseline vs over the course of the study) in predicting looking into exercise or fitness training.

Because our definition of engagement with health and wellness supports and services (i.e., the summary HSSQ scores across all assessment periods over the course of the study) was rather liberal, we reran HSSQ analyses with a more conservative definition of engagement as the HSSQ score obtained at the final assessment. At the final assessment, respondents were asked to report only about the time since their last assessment (ie, over the past 4–6 months). Supporting our findings with the liberal indicator, being in the VFBA group was associated with a significantly steeper increase in both looking into and receiving mindfulness and music training than being in the Control group. Also supporting our findings with the liberal indicator, being in the VFBA group was associated with a significantly steeper increase in looking into psychotherapy than being in the Control group (the difference approached statistical significance for receiving psychotherapy). In addition to replicating the above findings with the liberal indicator, we found that being in the VFBA group was associated with significantly steeper increases in looking into sleep-related services and in services addressing problems of living.

DISCUSSION

The VFBA was accepted in a primary care pediatrics setting. Pediatric practitioners and support staff joined the research team in developing the research protocol. Pediatric practitioners referred their patients and families to the study, and it ran continuously at UVM Pediatrics for more than 2 years. That practitioners referred their patients to the study was critical for this project, because researchers are not allowed to directly present interventional research opportunities to patients at the UVM MC. This project would have not been possible without the collaboration of the authors' pediatric colleagues.

Involvement of the pediatric practitioners and support staff in designing the protocol was key to assuring their engagement with the project. Because the primary care pediatric environment is intensive, it was important to develop study procedures that did not interfere with clinic operations or place demands on the clinic staff.

Family Wellness Coaches performed several functions in relation to families (ie, intervention, case management, health education, and care navigation), which could have been confusing to parents. However, parents understood the role played by

Family Wellness Coaches well, and responded positively to coaches. On average, parents had 36 contacts with Family Wellness Coaches over the course of the study.

Results also suggested that parents used a variety of modalities to communicate with Family Wellness Coaches. Only approximately a third of their contacts occurred face-to-face, with the rest occurring via e-mail, text messages, phone, or videoconferencing. The majority of Family Wellness Coaches' contacts with families occurred via e-mail and text messages (52%), indicating that Family Wellness Coaches need to be technically competent and technologically equipped to successfully engage families.

The topics that Family Wellness Coaches addressed in their interactions with families indicated their fidelity to the VFBA. The 5 most frequently addressed topics of exercise, mindfulness, child emotional and behavioral health, assessment of emotional and behavioral health, and music education suggested that Family Wellness Coaches consistently worked with families on wellness and on the monitoring of emotional and behavioral health, in accordance with the VFBA model.

Furthermore, the RCT design allowed rigorously testing the effect of the VFBA on family engagement with health and wellness supports and services. In comparison to pediatric care as usual, receiving the VFBA intervention was associated with a sharper increase in engagement with exercise/fitness, mindfulness, and music training and psychotherapy over the course of the study. This was true for both looking into and actually receiving these supports and services. These findings also indirectly supported the fidelity of the VFBA intervention offered in this study, because the VFBA emphasizes exercise, mindfulness, and music training due to the well-established positive effects of these activities on emotional and behavioral health.[3,4]

Finally, the findings indicated that the VFBA may be associated somewhat differently with the dispositional and behavioral aspects of engagement: The effects of the VFBA on looking into versus actually receiving health and wellness supports and services were not identical. Different definitions of engagement vis-à-vis the study timeline (ie, liberal vs conservative) showed different associations with the VFBA intervention. Developing a more nuanced understanding of family engagement, including its multifaceted nature and dynamics, could inform the development of the VFBA.

Results of this study need to be examined in the context of its limitations. Because this was an institutionally funded, pilot RCT that focused on feasibility and instrumentation, this study was small. The demonstrated feasibility of its procedures and the encouraging results, however, support the generalizability and upscaling of this research. Another limitation is that measurement of engagement with health and wellness supports and services could have confounded engagement with the availability of these supports and services to families. As a progressive city in a progressive state, Burlington offers an impressive array of social supports and services to families with children, and the state of Vermont offers free health insurance to all uninsured children in poverty. Therefore, although it cannot be ruled out, lack of availability was unlikely. Finally, results presented in this article do not address the effect of the VFBA on the health and well-being of the children and parents. This article was prepared weeks after the ending of the trial while the data set was being finalized. Reports on the health-related effects of the VFBA are forthcoming from our group.

Overall, the findings supported the feasibility of the VFBA in a primary care pediatric clinic and offered promising evidence of its effectiveness at engaging families in a variety of health and support services. The VFBA is an innovative approach to healthcare delivery that addresses several formidable challenges of the current healthcare system in the United States. The authors plan to continue developing it in response to the findings of this trial and to test it with greater rigor in larger RCTs.

REFERENCES

1. Barr A. Introduction to U.S. health policy: the organization, financing, and delivery of health care in America. 4th edition. Baltimore (MD): Johns Hopkins University Press; 2016.
2. Squires D, Anderson C. U.S. Health care from a global perspective: spending, use of services, prices, and health in 13 countries. Issue Brief (Commonw Fund) 2015;15:1–15.
3. Hudziak JJ, Ivanova MY. The Vermont Family Based Approach: family based health promotion, illness prevention, and intervention. Child Adolesc Psychiatr Clin N Am 2016;25(2):167–78.
4. Hudziak JJ, Bartels M. Genetic and environmental influences on wellness, resilience, and psychopathology: a family based approach for promotion, prevention, and intervention. In: Hudziak JJ, editor. Psychopathology and wellness: genetic and environmental influences. Arlington (VA): American Psychiatric Publishing; 2008. p. 267–86.
5. Denham SA. Relationships between family rituals, family routines, and health. J Fam Nurs 2003;9(3):305–30.
6. Christensen P. The health-promoting family: a conceptual framework for future research. Soc Sci Med 2004;59(2):377–87.
7. Prince M, Patel V, Saxena S, et al. No health without mental health. Lancet 2007; 370(9590):859–77.
8. Roehrig C. Mental disorders top the list of the most costly conditions in the United States: $201 billion. Health Aff 2016;35(6):1130–5.
9. Edelman CL, Kudzma EC. Health promotion throughout the life span. 9th edition. St Louis (MO): Elsevier; 2018.
10. United States Census Bureau. Quick facts: Burlington city, Vermont. Suitland (MD): United States Census Bureau; 2017. Available at: https://www.census.gov/quickfacts/fact/table/burlingtoncityvermont/PST045217. Accessed September 24, 2018.
11. Hollinshead AB. Four-factor index of social status. Unpublished manuscript. New Haven, CT: Yale University; 1975.
12. Achenbach TM. General description of 1975 Hollingshead occupational categories updated to 2001. Burlington (VT): Research Center for Children, Youth, and Families; 2002.

The University of Vermont Wellness Environment

Feasibility and Initial Results of a College Undergraduate Health-Promoting Program

Yang Bai, PhD[a], William E. Copeland, PhD[b], Zoe Adams, BS[c],
Matthew Lerner, PhD[c], Jessica A. King, MA[c], Steve Szopinski, MS[d],
Vinay Devadanam, BS[d], Jeff Rettew, PhD[d], Jim Hudziak, MD[e,*]

KEYWORDS

- Audit • DAST-10 • PHQ-9 • College students • Wellness • Behavior change
- Substance use

KEY POINTS

- The University of Vermont Wellness Environment is a neuroscience-inspired, incentive-based behavioral change program developed to promote well-being and prevent negative outcomes in college age students.
- It is feasible to collect high-quality data including daily surveys on college students in this program related to key outcomes, including drug and alcohol use, health-promoting behaviors, academic performance, and continued enrollment/retention.
- Over the course of an academic year, participation in both periodic and daily surveys were high, suggesting a full evaluation of the Wellness Environment program is a reasonable goal.
- According to institutional data provided by the University of Vermont Student Affairs, students living in the Wellness Environment residential hall during the 2017 to 2018 academic year had 81% fewer alcohol/drug incidents and 46% fewer student conduct violations than students living in typical residence halls.

Disclosure Statement: Dr J. Hudziak receives research grants from the Conrad Hilton Foundation and Apple Corp. for this work.
[a] Department of Rehabilitation and Movement Science, University of Vermont, Rowell 305, Burlington, VT 05401, USA; [b] Division of Child Psychiatry, Department of Psychiatry, Vermont Center for Children, Youth, and Families, University of Vermont, UHC St Joseph 3210A, 1 South Prospect Street, Burlington, VT 05401, USA; [c] Division of Child Psychiatry, Department Psychiatry, Vermont Center for Children, Youth, and Families, University of Vermont, 1 South Prospect Street, Room 3213, Burlington, VT 05401, USA; [d] Division of Student Affairs, University of Vermont, 1 South Prospect Street, Burlington, VT 05401, USA; [e] Division of Child Psychiatry, Department of Psychiatry, Vermont Center for Children, Youth, and Families, University of Vermont, 1 South Prospect Street, Burlington, VT 05401, USA
* Corresponding author.
E-mail address: James.Hudziak@uvm.edu

Child Adolesc Psychiatric Clin N Am 28 (2019) 247–265
https://doi.org/10.1016/j.chc.2018.11.011
1056-4993/19/© 2018 Elsevier Inc. All rights reserved.

Abbreviations	
ASR	adult self report
AUDIT	alcohol use disorders identification test
CIT	comprehensive inventory of thriving
DAST-10	drug abuse screening test
GPA	grade point average
MAAS	mindfulness attention awareness scale'
PHQ-9	patient health questionnaire
UVM WE	university of vermont wellness environment
WE APP	UVM WE mobile application

INTRODUCTION

The development of the adolescent brain has been the focus of a great deal of recent scientific inquiry. A number of scholars have drawn attention to the fact that the transitional age (teenage years to 25 years of age) brain may undergo a second critical period of development.[1] The neuroscience behind this idea is often called the developmental mismatch of adolescence.[2,3] The transitional age brain is undergoing a critical period of organization during which early maturation of subcortical regions (eg, amygdala, nucleus accumbens) are mismatched with still-developing regulatory prefrontal cortical regions.[1] At the same time, that transition-aged youth and their maturing brains need more external regulatory support and lower risk environments, they are often leaving home and entering college, where they have easier access to alcohol and drugs, high-risk social activities, and loss of close parenting and supervision. In contrast with the insufficient scaffolding that characterizes a stereotypical undergraduate experience, the University of Vermont Wellness Environment (UVM WE) program offers a neuroscience inspired, incentive-based behavioral change system designed to increase health-promoting behaviors and decrease substance misuse and abuse, as well as emotional and behavioral problems among transitional age college students with an overarching goal of improving academic performance and seeding life-long healthy habits.

In many ways, the developmental mismatch between cortical and subcortical structures and the pressures of the modern world on developing brains combine to create a perfect storm for negative health outcomes. For instance, national data suggest that adolescence and young adulthood are the developmental periods of greatest risk for developing substance abuse behaviors as well as a broad range of other high-risk behaviors, including criminality and risky sexual behavior.[4–6] These problems often contribute to a wide array of maladaptive behaviors, such as poor school performance, high rates of alcohol and other substance abuse, school dropout, property damage, physical and sexual assault, accidental injury, and suicidal behavior.[7–9] With all of these factors in play, it is not surprising that many teenagers and young adults suffer so mightily when they go to college. Findings from longitudinal studies of changes in the brain structure from childhood to adolescence and throughout the transitional years[10–12] indicate that neurodevelopmental processes, including pruning and increasing specialization, underlie the exquisite sensitivity of the transitional age brain to environmental influences. On one hand, the plasticity—and resulting resilience—of the transitional age brain provide a sensitive period during which the positive effects of health-promoting environmental influences are amplified. On the other hand, the same plasticity makes transitional age brains especially susceptible to harmful environmental influences. For instance, 5-year graduation rates for undergraduate students hover around 50%, and more than 1 million college students suffer from the sequelae of alcohol and other drug use. Therefore, it is imperative that new models of health promotion and illness prevention be developed for young brains in college.[13]

In response to this challenge, one of the authors (J.H.) designed, developed, implemented, and tested a neuroscience-inspired, incentivized behavioral change program at the UVM called the WE.[13] The goal was relatively straightforward: design a model college experience based on what is known about transitional age brain development, the negative impact of high-risk behaviors in a high-risk environment (eg, free of parental supervision and guidance), and emerging behavioral change and neuroimaging research. By improving decision making; providing knowledge, skills, and attitudes about the impact of one's choices on brain health; and using the power of choosing to engage in health-promoting activities over risky behaviors, the UVM WE program is hypothesized to improve health and academic outcomes by incentivizing behaviors that promote positive brain health and decrease normative risk for alcohol and drug use in college students.

THE UNIVERSITY OF VERMONT WELLNESS ENVIRONMENT DESIGN

The UVM WE program is rooted in the developmental neuroscience literature and rests on 4 pillars: physical fitness, nutrition, mindfulness, and interpersonal relationships (**Fig. 1**). Activities consistent with each pillar are implemented at 3 interrelated levels: didactic, residential, and app-based incentivized participation, guidance, and tracking in health-promoting activities.

The cornerstone of the didactic level of the UVM WE program is the course Healthy Brains, Healthy Bodies: Surviving and Thriving in College, in which students are taught the impact of specific behaviors on genomic (epi) and brain health (neuroplasticity) in a

Pillars of WE

Layers of Intervention		Nutrition	Mindfulness	Fitness	Relate
	Healthy Brains, Healthy Bodies	Gut-Brain Connection	Neuroscience of Mindfulness and Yoga	Neuroscience of Exercise	Neuroscience of Relationships
	Residential Halls	Dorm Snacks CCRH Dining Hall In-house Cooking Classes	In-house Yoga Mindfulness Events	In-house Gym Fitness On Demand In-house Pelaton bikes Incentivized Fitness Passes WE 420 5k	WE Mentors WE Mentor Events
	WE App	Log Water and Meals WE Coin Incentive for Logging Food	Yoga and Mindfulness Library	Exercise Library Log Workouts/Track Fitness WE Coin Incentive for Exercise	WE Coin Incentive for attending Events WE Event Calendar

Fig. 1. Wellness Environment (WE) design diagram. (*Courtesy of* J. Hudziak, MD, Burlington, VT.)

nonjudgmental context. The central theme of the course is that an individual's environment and choices impact on the function of the genome through epigenetic modifications, which in turn impact the structure and function of the brain and subsequent thoughts, beliefs, and behaviors. The course is designed to demonstrate that all health, emotional, general medical, cognitive, and academic outcomes are directly influenced by the thoughts, beliefs, and behaviors of the individual. By demonstrating that connection, this course provides the underlying rationale for the UVM WE program. In addition to this course, UVM students have the opportunity to continue studying the impact of health-promoting (and risky) behaviors on both brain development and overall health by completing a minor in Behavioral Change Health Studies. Example courses from the minor include: Your Brain on Drugs, The Science of Happiness, Living Behavioral Change, Family Wellness Coaching, and The Effects of Adversity.

The residential aspect of the WE design is an experiential extension and tangible application of the principles studied in the didactic component (ie, the 4 pillars of wellness). For instance, students in the residential community engage in brain-building wellness activities including incentivized daily exercise with personal trainers, music lessons, mindfulness and yoga with certified instructors, and healthy dietary practices under the guidance of a nutrition coach whose work is informed by recent advances in gut–brain neuroscience. Examples of how these behaviors are incentivized include the following. All WE students group and in house fitness passes are paid for up front (cost per student $260) and remain cost free as long as they use the passes a total of 40 times per year. If the student only uses the facility 20 times, they are required to pay back 50% of the upfront costs. Additionally, and discussed elsewhere in this article, on the WE App is a cryptocurrency, entitled WE Coin, that students earn by participation in wellness activities; for example, each time the student uses the gym they earn 50 WE coins. Thus, through incentivized, first-hand experience, students learn the impacts of hydration, sleep, and learning to play an instrument on their developing brains. Students also participate in WE Relate programming to better understand how to honor themselves, live in an affirmative environment, and engage in acts of kindness and gratitude. As an extension of the WE Relate programming, a mentoring program called WE Mentors was developed (www.wementor.org) to encourage participating undergraduates to provide guidance to local elementary school students and to mentor these children in activities that advance their personal wellness. Students who live in the WE are required to sign a contract that indicates they understand that if they have alcohol, drugs, or paraphernalia, or are grossly intoxicated in the WE, they will be removed from the program (and live elsewhere on campus). During the first full year of the WE App Research Study (2017–18), 15 students were required to transfer from the WE to other campus housing in response to violations of the policy prohibiting alcohol and drugs in the WE. After enthusiastic endorsement from university leadership, the program opened during the 2015 to 2016 school year with 120 students. The program grew to 480 students for the 2016 to 2017 academic year and to 806 for the 2017 to 2018 academic year.

The third aspect of the UVM WE program is the UVM WE mobile application (WE App). The WE App was designed to support student participation in daily health-promoting activities. To that end, students can use the WE app to set goals, check their progress, and receive incentives for engaging in health promotion activities. The WE App includes meditations specifically developed for college students, personalized yoga instruction through video education, and mentored physical fitness training exercises custom-made for college students. In addition, there includes a logging feature for a variety of health-promoting behaviors, including fitness, nutrition, sleep, and hydration. Most importantly, there is a nightly self-report survey that asks the students about their day by querying 14 items, 7 health-promoting related behaviors, 6 risk-related behaviors, and whether or not they had a happy, okay, or sad day. These data are archived for the student, allowing them at any time to review what their behaviors were on their happy, okay, or sad days and thus inform their personalized health planning. All of the health promoting activities, including the nightly survey are incentivized through a WE cryptocurrency called WE Coin. Each time a student logs engaging in a health-promoting activity, they have the opportunity to earn WE Coin. WE Coin is then stored within the WE App, in the WE Bank. Students can then use the WE Coin in the WE Store to purchase a variety of rewards (eg, outdoor experiences, bike passes, meals at local restaurants, clothing, exercise gear). For the 2017 to 2018 academic year, the approximate cost of providing rewards in the WE Store was $40,000. The current development version of the WE App can be used on both an Apple iPhone and Apple Watch; however, a future version will be compatible with both Apple and Android operating systems.

Finally, the UVM WE program has an aggressive research component built around 3 extensive questionnaire sessions conducted at the beginning (ie, baseline; the focus of this report), middle, and end of the academic year. From the beginning, assessment has been a core feature of the WE program, with information collected at regular intervals (baseline, midyear, and end of year) as well as daily. In addition to the periodic questionnaires, students complete a nightly 14-item health and risk survey on the WE App. The daily survey was developed for use in the WE App Study and can be seen in **Box 1**. To examine the effects of the WE program, typical university aggregate data such as grade point average (GPA), alcohol and drug abuse violations, and school retention are integrated with individual-level data from the periodic questionnaires and daily surveys.

This analysis presents baseline data collected at the beginning of the 2017 to 2018 academic year and focuses specifically on self-reported drug abuse, alcohol abuse, wellness-related behaviors, and emotional health symptoms, as well as university-level data on alcohol- and drug-related incidents and student retention. This analysis also shows that it is possible to collect daily survey data throughout the year on a broad range of health and wellness indicators using an iPhone or Apple Watch app. This article is not a formal evaluation of the entire WE program, but the current findings suggest that such an evaluation can be rigorous and include novel data collection efforts.

SAMPLE

All participants were recruited during the 2017 to 2018 academic year via an institutional review board-approved research protocol to test the impact of the UVM WE program and the WE App on college students' health behaviors and academic achievement. A total of 1941 students consented to participate, but 81 of those students were excluded because they failed to complete the initial battery of questionnaires, which resulted in 1860 students who agreed to participate, including 806 WE students and 1054 college as usual students (non-WE; **Fig. 2**). This sample is best considered a convenience sample of current UVM students. The rapid growth in student participation in the WE (ie, 120 in year 1, 480 in year 2, and 806 in year 3) suggests a strong interest among UVM students. All participants completed an informed consent approved by the UVM Institutional Review Board. All participating students in both conditions received a Series 1 Apple Watch that was used to collect the nightly survey data and encouraged health promotion through daily reminders to exercise and be active.

Box 1
Daily survey

1. How many hours of sleep did you get?
   Answers: 0, 1 to 3, 4 to 7, 8+

2. How many minutes did you exercise?
   Answers: 0, 1 to 30, 31 to 60, 61+

3. How many servings of fruit/vegetables did you eat?
   Answers: 0, 1 to 3, 4+

4. How many bottles of water did you have?
   Answers: 0, 1 to 3, 4 to 6, 7+

5. How many minutes have you practiced mindfulness?
   Answers: 0, 1 to 9, 10 to 30, 31+

6. How many minutes did you play an instrument or sing today?
   Answers: 0, 1 to 30, 31 to 60, 61+

7. How was your day?
   Answers: sad, okay, happy

8. How many hours did you spend non-academic screen time?
   Answers: 0, 1 to 2, 3 to 6, 7+

9. How many drinks did you have?
   Answers: 0, 1 to 2, 3 to 4, 5+

10. How many shots of liquor did you have?
    Answers: 0, 1 to 2, 3 to 4, 5+

11. How many times did you smoke/use marijuana?
    Answers: 0, 1 to 3, 4+

12. How many cigarettes did you smoke?
    Answers: 0, 1 to 3, 4+

13. How many times did you take illicit drugs?
    Answers: 0, 1 to 3, 4+

14. How many prescription pills (not yours) did you take?
    Answers: 0, 1 to 3, 4+

ASSESSMENT

Information on student functioning and relevant outcomes was collected in 2 ways: (1) a periodic battery of questionnaires to assess in-depth functioning and (2) daily surveys administered using the participants' mobile devices (ie, iPhone or Apple Watch) to assess within-individual variability in key outcomes (**Fig. 3**).

Periodic Questionnaires

To remain an active participant in the study, all participants were asked to complete 3 online self-report questionnaires throughout the 2017 to 2018 academic year. These self-report questionnaires were administered at baseline, midyear, and the end of the year through the online platform Campus Labs. The measures included in the questionnaire sets were: The Big Five Inventory,[14] Adult Self Report (ASR),[15] Brief Problem Monitor,[16] Screening Brief Intervention and Referral to Treatment, the WE Inventory of Thriving,[17,18] Mindfulness Attention Awareness Scale (MAAS),[19] Short Form Health Survey,[20] Alcohol Use Disorders Identification Test (AUDIT),[21] Drug Abuse

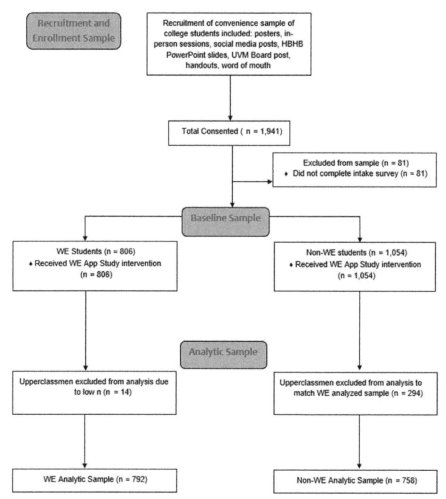

Fig. 2. CONSORT diagram of the Wellness Environment (WE) app study sample. (*Courtesy of* J. Hudziak, MD, Burlington, VT.)

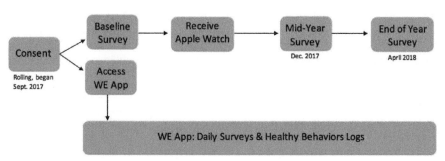

Fig. 3. Wellness Environment (WE) App Study participant flowchart for the 2017 to 2018 academic year. (*Courtesy of* J. Hudziak, MD, Burlington, VT.)

Screening Test (DAST-10)[22], and Patient Health Questionnaire (PHQ-9).[23] The ASR was administered at baseline and at the end of the year, and the Brief Problem Monitor was administered at midyear and the end of the year. All other measurements were collected at all 3 time points. Questionnaire data included information on alcohol and drug use, psychological health, mindfulness, level of thriving, personality, and a self-report measure of overall health (HSQ Short Form Health Survey[20]).

A detailed description of the substance abuse measures, mental health measures (AUDIT, DAST-10 and PHQ-9) and other additional measures is provided herein.

Adult Self Report

The ASR[18] is a nationally normed self-report instrument that provides dimensional information about 6 areas of an individual's level of adaptive function (personal strengths; friends; family; spouse/partner; job; education), symptoms of 8 empirically derived syndromes (anxious/depressed, withdrawn, attention problems, aggressive behavior, rule-breaking behavior, intrusiveness, somatic complaints, thought problems), and symptoms of 6 *Diagnostic and Statistical Manual of Mental Disorders*–oriented scales (eg, depressive problems, avoidant personality problems, antisocial personality problems). This measure yields scores and percentile ranks (with corresponding cutoff scores for clinical significance) on each subscale that are nationally normed by sex, within each of 2 age bands (18–35 or 36–59 years), based on nationally representative samples of adults. Given the close correspondence between the scales of the ASR those of the Child Behavior Checklist,[19] this measure can be particularly useful when examining similarities and differences between individuals within a family system.

The Big Five Index

The Big Five Index[20] is a self-report measure created to capture the dimensions of the Big Five model of personality.[21] This instrument includes 44 affirmative statements, each of which begins "I see myself as someone who. . . ." (eg, ". . . is talkative; is reserved"). Participants are asked to rate each item on a scale of 1 (disagree strongly) to 6 (agree strongly). Between 8 and 10 items are intended to represent each dimension of the Big Five model, and evidence from confirmatory factor models is consistent with this intended structure. Item-scale reliability coefficients range from 0.80 (neuroticism) to 0.92 (extroversion).

Brief Problem Monitor

The Brief Problem Monitor[22] comprises a subset of items from the ASR (described elsewhere in this article) and yields nationally normed, dimensional scores for internalizing, externalizing, attention problems, and total problems. This instrument can be used for self- or other-report. Scores on each scale can be compared with specific norms based on age, gender, and cultural group. Based on each set of norms, T-scores of 65 or greater (corresponding with the 93rd percentile in that individual's reference group) indicate cause for clinical concern.

Health Survey Questionnaire

The Health Survey Questionnaire,[23] the Short Form 36, is a self-report measure of overall health. This instrument comprises 36 questions and is designed for use in community settings. Items are designed to provide information about 8 areas of general health: physical functioning, social functioning, physical problems, emotional problems, pain, mental health, vitality, and general health perception. Scores across these dimensions are aggregated using an algorithm and scaled from 0 to 100, with higher scores indicating better health states.

Mindful Attention Awareness Scale

The MAAS[24] is a self-report measure of trait mindfulness. This instrument comprises 15 first-person statements (eg, "I could be experiencing some emotion and not be conscious of it until some time later" "I find myself listening to someone with one ear, doing something else at the same time") and provides response options ranging from 1 (almost always) to 6 (almost never) for each item. Total score on this measure is the average rating across all items, with lower scores indicating higher levels of mind-fulness. The MAAS was originally tested in 14 independent samples of college students (2277 total participants; mean, 3.83; standard deviation, 0.70). Subsequent evaluations of the MAAS have reported excellent psychometric properties, including a unitary factor structure and high levels of internal consistency (αs of 0.80–0.90[24,25]).

Wellness Environment Inventory of Thriving

The WIT was created as an adaptation of the Comprehensive Inventory of Thriving (CIT[26]) for use with participants in the WE. The CIT is a self-report measure of overall well-being that includes 7 subscales (relationship support, engagement, mastery, au-tonomy, meaning, optimism, and subjective well-being). The CIT was initially devel-oped with a sample of college students (n = 490) and later cross-validated in a series of 4 independent community samples (2701 total participants). Across samples, the CIT subscales demonstrated adequate to high internal consistency (αs of 0.71–0.96), and results of confirmatory factor models indicated that the proposed 7-factor structure fit the data well. In the original cross-validation sample, the addition of CIT scores to regression models predicting physical health outcomes provided significant incremental value, beyond predictions based on narrower thriving scales and beyond predictions based on anxiety and depression symptoms. In addition to 10 items taken directly or with only word-level edits from the CIT, the WIT includes 9 novel items intended to represent gratitude, mindfulness, exercise, sleep, and nutrition. The WIT comprises 20 declarative statements (eg, "The way I exercise has a positive impact on my well-being") with 3 response options (1 [disagree]; 2 [neither agree nor disagree]; 3 [agree]). Higher scores on the WIT are indicative of higher levels of well-being (**Fig. 4**).

Alcohol Use Disorders Identification Test

The AUDIT is a measure of behaviors associated with increased risk for harmful con-sequences of alcohol use.[21] Participants are asked to respond to 10 questions that address alcohol consumption, symptoms of dependence, and interpersonal conse-quences of alcohol use. Although it was originally developed for use with adults, inde-pendent research groups in the United States and other countries have reported adequate psychometric properties of the AUDIT when administered to undergraduate students.[24,25] Results of a study that compared AUDIT scores and diagnoses of alcohol use disorders based on semistructured face-to-face interviews in a sample of 251 undergraduate students (mean age, 20.56 years; standard deviation, 1.86 years; 46.8% female) indicated that a cut score of 6 for males or 3 for females was associated with a 97% sensitivity (but only 37% and 17% specificity, respectively).[26] Despite some limitations with regard to specificity, the sensitivity of the AUDIT is consistently high across studies, especially when used with undergraduates who are not seeking treatment for alcohol-related problems.

Please indicate your agreement or disagreement with each of the following statements using the scale below:

	Disagree	Neither Agree nor Disagree	Agree
1. There are people who appreciate me as a person	1	2	3
2. I am achieving most of my goals	1	2	3
3. I can succeed if I put my full effort into something	1	2	3
4. What I do in life matters	1	2	3
5. My life has a clear sense of purpose	1	2	3
6. My life is going well	1	2	3
7. I feel good most of the time	1	2	3
8. My sleep pattern has a positive impact on my life	1	2	3
9. I practice mindfulness in a way that has a positive impact on my well-being	1	2	3
10. The food I eat has a positive impact on my well-being	1	2	3
11. I feel a sense of belonging in my community	1	2	3
12. The way I exercise has a positive impact on my well-being	1	2	3
13. The way I show and experience appreciation for the world have a positive impact on my well-being	1	2	3
14. In most things I do, I feel energized	1	2	3
15. The amount of water I drink has a positive impact on my well-being	1	2	3
16. The way I handle stress has a positive impact on my well-being	1	2	3
17. I am confident that I can handle stressful situations	1	2	3
18. I am able to adjust to changes in my life	1	2	3
19. I am optimistic about my future	1	2	3
20. No matter what kind of person I am, I can always grow and change substantially	1	2	3

Fig. 4. Wellness inventory of thriving. (*Adapted from* Su R, Tay L, Diener E. The development and validation of the comprehensive inventory of thriving (CIT) and the brief inventory of thriving (BIT). Appl Psychol Health Well Being 2014;6(3):278–79; with permission.)

Drug Abuse Screening Test

The DAST is a quantitative self-report instrument designed to measure maladaptive use of psychoactive substances during the past 12 months.[22] Responses on each of 10 yes/no items are scored 1 or 0, yielding a total score between 0 and 10. Although the DAST is a quantitative instrument designed to provide dimensional measurement of substance abuse, findings are consistent with the use of a cut score of 3 on the 10-item version as a predictor of diagnostic status. For instance, compared with diagnoses based on the combination of semistructured interviews and urinalysis, using a cut score of 3, the DAST-10 was found to correctly distinguish between individuals with and without a substance abuse problem in 93% of cases.[27]

Patient Health Questionnaire

The PHQ-9 is a quantitative self-report measure that maps directly onto the 9 *Diagnostic and Statistical Manual of Mental Disorders,* 5th edition, symptoms of a major depressive episode.[23] This instrument allows respondents to report both the number of symptoms present and the severity of each symptom. Each of 9 items (eg, "Little interest or pleasure in doing things," "Poor appetite or overeating") is scored on a 4-point scale ranging from 0 (not at all) to 3 (nearly every day). The possible range of scores is 0 to 27. This measure shows high internal consistency ($\alpha = 0.89$) and corresponds well with diagnoses made on the basis of a standard diagnostic interview. Scores on the PHQ-9 correspond closely (ie, $r = 0.81$) with scores on the 21-item Beck Depression Inventory-II, especially in community settings.[28]

Daily Surveys

All participants in the study were provided with a Series 1 Apple Watch (as described elsewhere in this article) and asked to download and use the WE App developed by Dr Hudziak. In addition, participants were asked to complete daily surveys administered through the WE App or Apple Watch. The daily survey was open from 7:00 PM to 11:59 PM every evening and prompted participants to consider their health- and wellness-related behaviors throughout the day. Data collected from the WE App included 14 health- and risk-related behaviors (ie, cigarette use, consumption of alcoholic drinks, minutes of exercise, illicit drug use, shots of liquor, minutes of mindfulness, mood, minutes of music played/sang, nutrition, number of prescription pills, hours of sleep, marijuana use, hours of technology, and amount of water consumed). For example, the item used to measure sleep is: "How many hours of sleep did you get?" Response options for this item are 0, 1 to 3, 4 to 7, and 8 hours or more (**Fig. 5**). The full text of this survey can be seen in **Box 1**.

STATISTICAL ANALYSIS

Descriptive statistics for demographic variables including gender, ethnicity, and year in college were computed separately for WE and non-WE students, and baseline group differences (WE vs non-WE) were examined using a χ^2 test. Completion rates for the periodic questionnaires (beginning, middle, end of the year) and daily surveys were also examined. The baseline scores for alcohol abuse, drug abuse, and depression symptoms from the AUDIT, DAST-10, and PHQ-9 were computed separately for WE and non-WE participants, and group mean differences were tested separately by gender, race/ethnicity, and year in school (ie, first- or second-year students). Daily survey data from October 2017 were used as the baseline measure. Participants who completed the survey on a minimum of 5 of 31 days were included in the analysis. The prevalence of health- and risk-related behaviors as reported in the daily surveys was calculated at the individual level first. Group means and group differences were then calculated and tested between WE and non-WE participants. All analyses were conducted with SAS 9.4 (Cary, NC) software. The alpha value for significance testing was set at 0.05.

RESULTS
Sample Description and Compliance

A total of 1941 participants were initially recruited. Eighty-one students who failed to complete baseline assessments were excluded from the current analysis. The resulting sample consists of 1860 participants, 1054 non-WE and 806 WE students who completed the baseline assessment. At the midpoint assessment, a total of 612 WE participants and 751 non-WE participants submitted the wave 2 questionnaires. The completion rate increased to 654 WE students and 833 non-WE students for the wave 3 questionnaires. A total of 745 control students and 602 WE students provided questionnaire data at all 3 time points (baseline, midyear, and end of the year). The characteristics of the participants who completed all baseline questionnaires are summarized in **Table 1**. Overall, more than two-thirds of participants enrolled in the WE App Study were female, regardless of group. Caucasian (88.6% and 85.7% for WE and non-WE participants, respectively) was the most prevalent ethnic group, followed

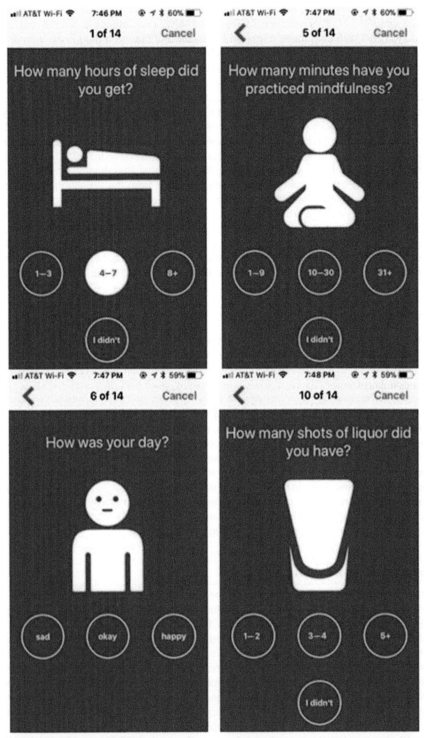

Fig. 5. Screenshot from the Wellness Environment (WE) app. (*Courtesy of* J. Hudziak, MD, Burlington, VT.)

Table 1					
Descriptive statistics of sample characteristics					
	WE		**Non-WE**		
	(N = 806)		**(N = 1054)**		
	n	**%**	**n**	**%**	**P**
Gender					
Female	573	71.8	686	65.3	<.05
Male	221	27.7	362	34.4	
Other	4	0.5	3	0.3	
Ethnicity					
African American	10	1.3	20	1.9	>.05
Asian	33	4.2	64	6.2	
Caucasian	702	88.6	890	85.7	
Latina/Latino	23	2.9	28	2.7	
Native American	4	0.5	1	0.1	
Pacific Islander	1	0.1	4	0.4	
Other	19	2.4	31	3.0	
Academic year					
First year of college	666	83.3	429	41.0	<.05
Second year of college	120	15.0	322	30.8	
Third year of college	14	1.8	240	22.9	
Fourth year of college	0	0	56	5.4	

Abbreviation: WE, wellness environment.
The number may not add up to total N owing to missing data in certain demographic questions.

sequentially by Asian, Latino, African American, Native American, Pacific Islander, and others. The Native American, Pacific Islander, and others comprised less than 5% of the sample. Thus, it was not possible to conduct WE versus non-WE comparisons specifically for these participants; however, all WE App Study participants are included in analyses of the full sample and comparisons not based on race/ethnicity (ie, male vs female; first- vs second-year students). Most of the WE participants were first-year college students (83.3%); the control participants were more equally distributed among first- (41%), second- (30.8%) and third-year (22.9%) students. Thus, to match the WE and non-WE participant populations, the subsequent analyses included only first- and second-year students. No group differences were found between WE and non-WE participants by race distribution, but statistically significant differences were found for gender and academic year distribution ($P<.05$).

Periodic Measures

Almost all students enrolled in this protocol provided baseline questionnaire data, and the data from the periodic battery focused on those students. **Table 2** shows the raw scores for alcohol abuse, drug abuse, and depression symptoms, computed separately for WE and non-WE participants at baseline. WE participants showed statistically significantly lower baseline scores for alcohol and drug abuse compared with non-WE participants among female, male, Caucasian, and first- and second-year students ($P<.05$). No statistically significant baseline differences were found for depression symptoms ($P>.05$).

Daily Surveys

A total of 850 non-WE and 682 WE participants provided daily survey data. In terms of participation rate, 359 WE participants (52.6%) and 491 non-WE participants (57.8%)

Table 2
The descriptive statistics of alcohol abuse, drug abuse, and depression scores by WE and control at baseline measured by AUDIT, DAST, and PHQ

	AUDIT			DAST			PHQ		
	WE	Non-WE	P	WE	Non-WE	P	WE	Non-WE	P
Gender									
Female	4.7 (4.3)	7.1 (4.5)	<.0001	0.8 (1.4)	1.0 (1.4)	.0041	6.7 (5.2)	6.2 (5.3)	.07
Male	5.6 (4.9)	8.3 (5.8)	<.0001	1.2 (1.9)	1.5 (1.7)	.0083	5.1 (5.1)	4.7 (4.6)	.39
Ethnicity									
African American	6.3 (5.5)	4.6 (5.2)	.35	1.3 (1.4)	0.4 (0.8)	.13	6.8 (6.3)	5.1 (3.9)	.38
Asian	2.5 (2.9)	4.0 (3.5)	.13	1.1 (2.1)	0.8 (1.2)	.46	6.8 (6.0)	5.8 (5.2)	.36
Caucasian	5.1 (4.5)	7.9 (5.0)	.0001	0.9 (1.5)	1.3 (1.6)	<.0001	6.2 (5.2)	5.7 (5.2)	.09
Latina/Latino	4.3 (4.2)	6.4 (5.3)	.05	0.7 (1.0)	1.0 (1.1)	.54	7.2 (4.8)	4.9 (4.0)	.11
Academic year									
Freshman	5.0 (4.5)	7.4 (5.2)	<.0001	0.9 (1.6)	1.3 (1.6)	<.0001	6.3 (5.2)	6.0 (5.3)	.43
Sophomore	4.8 (4.3)	7.5 (4.9)	<.0001	0.8 (1.6)	1.2 (1.5)	.0056	6.3 (5.7)	5.7 (5.0)	.23

Abbreviations: AUDIT, alcohol use disorders identification test; DAST, drug abuse screening test; PHQ, patient health questionnaire; WE, wellness environment.
Data are presented as mean (standard deviation).

completed at least 70% of the daily surveys during the 2017 to 2018 school year. A total of 460 WE participants (67.4%) and 628 non-WE participants (73.9%) completed at least 60% of the daily surveys, and 527 WE participants (77.3%) and 695 non-WE participants (81.8%) completed at least 50% of the daily surveys. The average number of total daily surveys completed per participant was 136 (out of a possible 209 days) with similar completion rates between WE and non-WE participants.

Table 3 shows the prevalence of self-reported health- and wellness-related behaviors by WE and non-WE participants in October 2017 as a baseline measure. The 593 WE participants and 499 non-WE participants who had at least 5 days of valid data in October are included in the analyses. WE participants had statistically significantly higher rates of sleeping more than 8 hours a day ($P = .04$), exercising more than 30 minutes per day ($P = .04$), consuming at least 1 serving of fruit or vegetable per day ($P = .0002$), and daily mindfulness practice ($P<.0001$). WE participants also had statistically significantly lower rates of engaging in drug and alcohol use or abuse behaviors including lower rates of (a) having at least 1 drink ($P<.0001$), (b) having at least 1 shot of liquor ($P<.0001$), (c) using marijuana at least once ($P<.0001$), (d) smoking at least 1 cigarette ($P<.0001$), (e) using illicit drugs at least once ($P = .0003$), and (f) taking at least 1 pill prescribed to another person ($P = .0002$) daily. No group differences were found between WE and non-WE students for the probability of playing an instrument, mood state, or having more than 3 hours of screen time ($P>.05$). These data are presented only to demonstrate the feasibility of collecting this type of data as well as potentially understanding the differences between the students who live in the WE and those who do not. We wish it to be clear that no causal comparisons can be made owing to the ascertainment bias inherent in the students' choice to live in or not live in the WE.

Institutional Data

Finally, the university maintains aggregate information on student academic achievement and disciplinary incidents. To maintain student confidentiality, this information is

Table 3
The prevalence of health- and wellness-related behaviors self-reported by WE and non-WE participants at baseline (October) measured by the WE App daily survey

	WE	Non-WE	P
Having a happy day	47.7% (26.5%)	45.9% (27.1%)	.26
Sleep >8 h/d	40.0% (26.1%)	36.8% (26.9%)	.04
Exercise >30 min/d	48.6% (28.8%)	45.0% (29.7%)	.04
Consume ≥1 serving of fruit and veggies/day	84.1% (21.4%)	79.0% (24.4%)	.0002
Having ≥4 bottles of water/day	50.89% (36.9%)	48.4% (36.8%)	.29
Having ≥1 drink/day	6.1% (9.7%)	14.3% (16.6%)	<.0001
Having ≥1 shots/d	5.1% (7.9%)	9.3% (13.4%)	<.0001
Having ≥1 marijuana/day	4.2% (12.8%)	12.9% (24.7%)	<.0001
Having ≥1 cigarettes/d	1.1% (6.4%)	4.0% (14.1%)	<.0001
Having ≥1 illicit drugs/d	0.3% (1.7%)	1.3% (6.9%)	.0003
Having ≥1 illicit pills/d	0.7% (4.0%)	2.3% (9.5%)	.0002
Practicing meditation ≥1 time/day	39.3% (26.4%)	28.6% (31.4%)	<.0001
Playing instrument or sing ≥1 time/day	47.2% (37.5%)	49.6% (37.3%)	.30
Spending ≥3 h of screen time/day	39.8% (31.0%)	39.4% (30.7%)	.84

Abbreviation: WE, wellness environment.
Screen time excludes academic screen time.

only available through the UVM Office of Student Affairs. According to findings provided by UVM Student Affairs, the WE residential hall had 0.84% alcohol/drug community standard incidents per student compared with 10.8% in the non-WE residential halls on campus in the 2017 to 2018 academic year. For alcohol/drug conduct violations, 46.0% fewer WE students were determined to be responsible after undergoing a full adjudication process, compared with non-WE students. Academic performance data from fall of 2017 also showed favorable results. WE students had a 90.0% retention rate compared with 85.0% among non-WE students, and WE students had a statistically significantly ($P<.05$) higher average GPA of 3.36 compared with 3.22 among non-WE students. Campus-wide alcohol use by students has decreased by 33.0% since the inception of the WE program, and the number of students requiring medical attention for excessive drinking at UVM has decreased by 50.0%. It must be noted that the dramatic decreases in campus-wide alcohol use and students requiring medical attention for excessive drinking is due to a wide number of initiatives started by the Division of Student Affairs and the Center for Health and Wellbeing at UVM before the creation of the WE program. Although it is possible that the WE program has contributed to these campus-wide reductions, it is impossible to tell.

Dissemination

The WE model has provided a roadmap for how to bring together multiple programs usually run by separate departments on campus. More than 70 different entities have contacted the WE for guidance and on how to further use aspects of the WE model.

Existing infrastructure and on-campus programs within higher education institutions provide the possibility to overcome the negative problems of the current college and university cultures. As our data mature, it may be possible to demonstrate that incentivized health promotion and prevention approaches may lead to improved overall college health and diminished consequences of alcohol and drug use and misuse, as well as the epidemic of emotional behavioral problems in college age students. Although most institutions have some programming in yoga/mindfulness, fitness, and mentoring, it is rarely programmatic and incentivized. One key challenge in replicating the WE model is securing high-level commitment at the university level to deliver resource allocation. The larger operational challenges lie in overcoming barriers between departments that subscribe to their individual norms with different frameworks, visions, and goals (eg, Campus Recreation, Psychiatry services, Student Affairs, class approval committees). Blending together resources and creating new requirements around a neuroscience-based approach requires participation from high levels of campus leadership. Establishing new leadership uniting faculty, residential life and other departments will necessarily give rise to challenges in service of bringing behavior change to a campus culture.

Institutional support and funding

A necessity for success is the need to build relationships through a campus champion, high-level faculty member, or administrator with the will and ability to keep developing and establishing the program foundation from which the WE model can flourish. Because this program has been funded from multiple cost centers, 3 major areas are identified in getting the program off the ground. First, staffing from the WE was funded from multiple sources at its outset, with the UVM Center for Health and Wellbeing, Larner College of Medicine, and Residential Life all contributing to the staff who delivered the program. As of 2017, the WE had 5 full-time staff devoted to programming, along with a number of individuals contributing to research, business operations, and course curriculum for the nearly 1200 students in the WE program. Next, funding for incentives available in the WE store came from the Residential Life programmatic funding, creating an early arrival program, WEventure, and the Conrad Hilton Fund Grant. Finally, the WE has received a number of donations from alumni and corporations interested in furthering this work. This support has been in the form of programmatic dollars to help fund Apple Watches, Peloton bikes, and incentives such as Burton clothing.

DISCUSSION

A core precis put forward by the creator of UVM WE program is that college students, if given the chance to make healthy decisions, will make healthy decisions. If college and universities are able to surround their students with opportunities and like-minded peers to engage in healthy brain building activities, they will. If, every time a student turns around, they have opportunities to engage in yoga, relationship building, acts of kindness and gratitude, fitness, mindfulness, healthy nutrition, and mentoring activities, they are likely to choose these activities. This fundamental precis is counterbalanced by the fact that, in many university and college residence halls and campuses, the student may turn around and be offered alcohol, cannabis, other drugs and high-risk behaviors, making the choice of wellness more difficult. The UVM WE program, although in its early stages, and only reliably tested in those students who live in the WE, has demonstrated that by offering and incentivizing wellness, students embrace it, and have better academic and behavioral outcomes and far less negative alcohol and conducts behaviors. Results from the 2017 to 2018 year of the WE confirm that the integrated educational, residential, and App-based facets of the WE programming can be implemented at a large scale and integrated with in-depth, multimodal data collection. Preliminary results at the institutional level, including higher GPA and retention as well as dramatically lower rates of alcohol and drug incidents among WE students, are promising but not causal, because the ascertainment bias cannot be ruled out. If longitudinal analyses reveal similar group differences, the WE would represent a promising health promotion and risk reduction intervention for college students. It is also possible that the results regarding group differences over the course of the year may be more modest than the institutional data would suggest. Even in that case, any significant decrease in substance abuse and conduct violations, along with any significant increase in nutrition, sleep, exercise, and GPA, would suggest that the WE can have a meaningful effect on the college environment. This question is the subject of ongoing analyses that will be reported separately.

Limitations

At baseline, there were preexisting differences between students who elected to live in the WE and those who did not, and these differences will be taken into account when examining the trajectory of risk- and health-related behaviors over the course of the 2017 to 2018 academic year. For the data from 2017 to 2018, we acknowledge that no causal, across sample, comparisons can be made. Our current database for the 2018 to 2019 academic year will allow us to test the impact of the WE environment in a more causal manner. There are many more freshmen at UVM this academic year (2018–2019) who selected WE as their primary signature program then could be included in the residential halls of WE. We currently have 760 freshmen who live in WE this year; of that number, 620 are enrolled in the study (the others do not have Apple phones or chose not to participate) and 600 non-WE students also enrolled in the study. At the end of this academic year, we will be able to perform classic comparison analyses between those students who live in WE, those who selected to live in WE but were placed in a learning community, and those who had no desire to live in WE. As long as some portion of the non-WE sample did not state a preference to live in the WE (ie, self-selection to non-WE), we expect to find similar baseline differences between WE and non-WE students. Going forward, these differences will be quantified and accounted for by implementing broader pretest assessments, collecting retrospective data, and increasing the size of the causally interpretable sample by increasing the use of random selection of WE students from the larger group who stated a preference to live in the WE yet live in a different learning community. In this way, we hope to disentangle program effects from preexisting baseline differences between WE and non-WE participants. Altogether, these data suggest that a full evaluation of the WE program integrating multimodal assessment methods is both feasible and warranted, given the preliminary evidence of improved academic outcomes and negative outcomes in both the WE students and the campus overall.

REFERENCES

1. Chung WW, Hudziak JJ. The transitional age brain: "the best of times and the worst of times". Child Adolesc Psychiatr Clin N Am 2017;26(2):157–75.
2. Giedd JN, Blumenthal J, Jeffries NO, et al. Brain development during childhood and adolescence: a longitudinal MRI study. Nat Neurosci 1999;2:861–3.
3. Giedd JN, Blumenthal J, Jeffries NO, et al. Development of the human corpus callosum during childhood and adolescence: a longitudinal MRI study. Prog NeuroPsychopharmacol Biol Psychiatry 1999;23:571–88.
4. Martins SS, Sarvet A, Santaella-Tenorio J, et al. Changes in US lifetime heroin use and heroin use disorder: prevalence from the 2001-2002 to 2012-2013 National Epidemiologic Survey on Alcohol and Related Conditions. JAMA Psychiatry 2017;74(5):445–55.
5. Dawson DA, Goldstein RB, Grant BF. Rates and correlates of relapse among individuals in remission from DSM-IV alcohol dependence: a 3-year follow-up. Alcohol Clin Exp Res 2007;31(12):2036–45.
6. Hasin DS, Kerridge BT, Saha TD, et al. Prevalence and correlates of DSM-5 cannabis use disorder, 2012-2013: findings from the national epidemiologic survey on alcohol and related conditions–III. Am J Psychiatry 2016;173(6):588–99.
7. Blanco C, Hasin DS, Wall MM, et al. Cannabis use and risk of psychiatric disorders: prospective evidence from a us national longitudinal study. JAMA Psychiatry 2016;73(4):388–95.
8. Erskine H, Moffitt T, Copeland W, et al. A heavy burden on young minds: the global burden of mental and substance use disorders in children and youth. Psychol Med 2015;45(07):1551–63.
9. Ferrari AJ, Norman RE, Freedman G, et al. The burden attributable to mental and substance use disorders as risk factors for suicide: findings from the Global Burden of Disease Study 2010. PLoS One 2014;9(4):e91936.
10. Giedd JN, Snell JW, Lange N, et al. Quantitative magnetic resonance imaging of human brain development: ages 4–18. Cereb Cortex 1996;6(4):551–9.
11. Giedd JN, Blumenthal J, Jeffries NO, et al. Brain development during childhood and adolescence: a longitudinal MRI study. Nat Neurosci 1999;2(10):861–3.
12. Gogtay N, Giedd JN, Lusk L, et al. Dynamic mapping of human cortical development during childhood through early adulthood. Proc Natl Acad Sci U S A 2004;101(21):8174–9.

13. Hudziak JJ, Tiemeier GL. Neuroscience-inspired, behavioral change program for university students. Child Adolesc Psychiatr Clin 2017;26(2):381–94.
14. John OP, Donahue EM, Kentle RL. The big five inventory–versions 4a and 54. Berkeley, CA: University of California, Berkeley; 1991.
15. Achenbach TM, Rescorla LA. Manual for the ASEBA adult forms & profiles. Burlington, VT: University of Vermont, Center for Children, Youth, & Families; 2003.
16. Achenbach TM, McConaughy SH, Ivanova MY, et al. Manual for the brief problem monitor. Burlington, VT: University of Vermont, Center for Children, Youth, & Families; 2018.
17. Su R, Tay L, Diener E. The development and validation of the comprehensive inventory of thriving (CIT) and the brief inventory of thriving (BIT). Appl Psychol Health Well Being 2014;6(3):251–79.
18. Rettew JH, Whitworth P. Manual for the wellness environment inventory of thriving. Burlington, VT: University of Vermont, Center for Children, Youth, & Families; 2016.
19. Brown KW, Ryan RM. The benefits of being present: mindfulness and its role in psychological well-being. J Pers Soc Psychol 2003;84(4):822–48.
20. Brazier JE, Harper R, Jones NM, et al. Validating the SF-36 health survey questionnaire: new outcome measure for primary care. BMJ 1992;305:160–4.
21. Babor TF, Biddle-Higgins JC, Saunders JB, et al. AUDIT: the alcohol use disorders identification test: guidelines for use in primary health care. In: AUDIT: the alcohol use disorders identification test: guidelines for use in primary health care. Geneva (Switzerland): World Health Organization; 2001.
22. Skinner HA. The drug abuse screening test. Addict Behav 1982;7:363–71.
23. Kroenke K, Spitzer RL, Williams JBW. The PHQ-9: validity of a brief depression severity measure. J Gen Intern Med 2001;16(9):606–13.
24. MacDonald R, Fleming M, Barry KL. Risk factors associated with alcohol abuse in college students. Am J Drug Alcohol Abuse 1991;4:439–49.
25. DeMartini KS, Carey KB. Optimizing the use of the AUDIT for alcohol screening in college students. Psychol Assess 2012;24(4):954–63.
26. Hagman BT. Performance of the AUDIT in detecting DSM-5 alcohol use disorders in college students. Subst Use Misuse 2016;51(11):1521–8.
27. Bohn MJ, Babor TF, Kranzler HR. Validity of the drug abuse screening test (DAST-10) in inpatient substance abusers: problems of drug dependence. Proceedings of the 53rd annual scientific meeting, The committee on problems of drug dependence, DHHS publication no. 92-1888. NIDA Research Monograph 1991;119:233.
28. Kung S, Alarcon RD, Williams MD, et al. Comparing the beck depression inventory-II (BDI-II) and Patient Health Questionnaire (PHQ-9) depression measures in an integrated mood disorders practice. J Affect Disord 2013;145:341–3.

Teaching Well-Being
From Kindergarten to Child Psychiatry Fellowship Programs

David C. Rettew, MD[a,b,c],*, Isaac Satz[d], Shashank V. Joshi, MD[e,f,g]

KEYWORDS

- Psychiatric training • Social-emotional learning • Science of happiness • Education
- Resiliency training

KEY POINTS

- Psychiatric training for medical students, residents, and fellows can integrate well-being principles to improve mental health.
- From preschool to college, principles of wellness and health promotion are increasingly prevalent and are showing promising results.
- Courses on happiness and well-being have been embraced at colleges and universities.
- Well-being is now a required component of child and adolescent psychiatry training.
- Training residents and fellows in emotional and behavioral well-being requires incorporation into clinical supervision and the overall culture and infrastructure of the training program.

INTRODUCTION

Psychiatric training at medical schools, residencies, and fellowships is heavily weighted toward the understanding and treatment of mental illness at the exclusion of more explicit teaching about well-being. Similarly, much of the mental health training for educators of children, adolescents, and young adults is directed toward

Disclosure Statement: The authors have no financial relationships to disclose.
[a] Department of Psychiatry, University of Vermont Larner College of Medicine, 1 South Prospect Street, Arnold 3, Burlington, VT 05401, USA; [b] Department of Pediatrics, University of Vermont Larner College of Medicine, 1 South Prospect Street, Arnold 3, Burlington, VT 05401, USA; [c] Child, Adolescent, and Family Unit, Vermont Department of Mental Health, 280 State Drive, NOB North, Waterbury, VT 05671, USA; [d] Swarthmore College, 500 College Avenue, Swarthmore, PA 19081, USA; [e] Department of Psychiatry, Stanford University School of Medicine, 401 Quarry Road, Room 1119, Stanford, CA 94305, USA; [f] Department of Pediatrics, Stanford University School of Medicine, 401 Quarry Road, Room 1119, Stanford, CA 94305, USA; [g] Graduate School of Education, Stanford University School of Medicine, 401 Quarry Road, Room 1119, Stanford, CA 94305, USA
* Corresponding author. 1 South Prospect Street, Arnold 3, Burlington, VT 05401.
E-mail address: David.rettew@med.uvm.edu

Child Adolesc Psychiatric Clin N Am 28 (2019) 267–280
https://doi.org/10.1016/j.chc.2018.11.007
1056-4993/19/© 2018 Elsevier Inc. All rights reserved.

the early identification and treatment of specific psychiatric symptoms. More recently, several initiatives across all levels of learning have taken place to specifically teach principles of well-being and techniques that can help individuals promote healthy brain development. To help future psychiatrists and child psychiatrists become experts not only in treating mental illness but also in promoting emotional-behavioral wellness, direct efforts are needed to teach these topics effectively.

For emotional-behavioral well-being to be fully incorporated into child psychiatry, it needs to be deliberately taught. Currently, most of the teaching in medical schools, general psychiatry residencies, and child psychiatry fellowships is directed at treating mental illness rather than promoting mental health. When students learn about depression, for example, it is rare that the educational content includes the topic of happiness. When trainees learn about abuse and maltreatment, there is usually little discussion about the positive parenting approaches that can help children thrive. Although there is no doubt that psychopathology remains deserving of rigorous study among the next generation of psychiatrists, the absence of specific education devoted to human well-being has been increasingly noticed and questioned. In response, there have recently been several efforts put forth to address this educational opportunity and to ensure that psychiatric training moving forward includes explicit teaching on emotional-behavioral well-being.

At the clinical level, these educational endeavors stand a better chance of gaining traction with children and their families if principles of wellness and health promotion have already been introduced and promoted earlier in life. From K12 education settings to college and postgraduate education, teachers and professors have increasingly understood their role to include the identification of mental illness among their students and the accommodation of psychiatric symptoms in their curricula. Many educators now also explicitly teach principles and techniques that promote emotional and behavioral well-being and principles of positive psychology with hopes of potentially inhibiting the onset of psychopathology.

As Suldo highlights,[1] the foundation for this work was laid decades before by Carl Rogers' person-centered approach to mental health, which focuses on an individual's self-actualizing tendencies. Rogers also was among the first to highlight how happiness can naturally develop from purposeful efforts to live fully and to strive toward reaching one's potential.[2] School-wide curricula geared toward cultivating social and emotional health among students in school settings, including connections with trusted adults, are termed under the broad category of social-emotional learning (SEL). Multiple resources for this approach are listed at www.casel.org/, and the site includes specific descriptions and existing empirical support for programs that have been found helpful in building skills for managing emotions, conveying empathy, making responsible decisions, and forming positive relationships.[1] Joshi and colleagues[3] have summarized how some of these SEL strategies can be practically applied as part of comprehensive health promotion and suicide prevention. This article summarizes some of the efforts underway toward the education of well-being and positive psychiatry principles at different levels of learning. Although the distinction between education and treatment/intervention can be muddled, the focus here is on efforts directed toward students in educational settings who are not specifically identified as suffering from mental disorders.

K12 EDUCATIONAL SETTINGS

Attention to well-being in schools is part of a prevention-oriented and resource-building approach to student education and mental health services. In high schools, emotional intelligence and well-being take on particular importance as rates of depression, anxiety, and various other mental health disorders are known to surge during this time.[4,5] The increased risk of psychopathology during this period coupled with a critical shortage of mental health professionals provides an opportunity for mental wellness and emotional intelligence-based curricula in the school setting to help students cope with stress and manage intense feelings. This collective curriculum-based approach is a relatively new idea, however, and the best methods for conveying the skills and knowledge needed to help students are still being discovered.

The assessment of a student's subjective well-being can allow school mental health providers to capture psychological wellness along the continuum of functioning, from severely distressed to content to fully thriving. A well-studied instrument is the SEHS (Social and Emotional Health Survey).[6] This tool assesses *covitality*, which can be conceptualized as the counterpart to *comorbidity*. It has been specifically described as "the synergistic effect of positive mental health resulting from the interplay among multiple positive-psychological building blocks."[7] A full description of the covitality construct is described in Furlong.[8]

Because high subjective well-being in students can serve protective functions,[9] whereas negative academic and health outcomes are associated with low subjective well-being (even in the absence of high-risk indicators for psychopathology), it becomes even more important to target student well-being specifically.[1,10] Empiric support for this approach is exemplified in a study of Australian high school students who were surveyed at multiple time points in the school year.[11] This study found that positive experiences at school promoted a greater positive affect overall. These benefits included aspects of school life that met students' psychological needs through feeling connected to teachers and peers, being confident in their academic abilities, and valuing their education overall. The resulting cheerful dispositions, in turn, facilitated more positive experiences at school. As Suldo writes in her summary of this research[1]:

> Thus, happiness was both an outcome and a cause of healthy experiences of relatedness, competence, and autonomy at school. These reciprocal relations demonstrated how students' positive affect can lead to an "upward spiral of positive school experiences and happiness over time (p239)."

In K12 settings, education about well-being can take many forms. Waters[12] has reviewed 5 different types of Positive Psychology Interventions (PPIs), based on Seligman's PERMA model (see McCormick in this issue for description of these 5 PERMA components), that can occur in schools to help students learn how to cultivate their own well-being. As shown in **Table 1**, these include programs and activities designed to enhance qualities such as hope, gratitude, and resilience. One example consists of each student writing down 3 good things that happened each day, whereas another involves completing a survey that assesses their particular character strengths.[13] The use of the gratitude visit, in which students compose and deliver a letter of thanks to someone who has helped them in the past, is another commonly used activity. These generally short exercises contain ideas and practices that can be applied beyond the classroom. Although not requiring large amounts of effort, they can exert real benefits on a student's perceived quality of life, which in turn is linked to academic performance.[13,14]

The various techniques and methods that are taught to enhance emotional intelligence and well-being have roots that stem from different traditions, most prominently positive psychology, mindfulness and meditation practices, and cognitive-behavioral therapy (CBT) oriented interventions. Each has its own potential benefits and

Table 1
Description of classroom well-being programs and exercises

Intervention	Applications and Program Descriptions

Interventions that focus on Hope	• Marques et al,[43] 2011
	  ○ 5-wk hope-based intervention program with middle schools students
	  ○ Students had significantly enhanced levels of hope, self-worth, and life satisfaction that persisted for 18 mo

Interventions that focus on Gratitude	• Froh et al,[44] (2008)
	  ○ Seventh, eighth, and ninth grade students recorded up to 5 things they were grateful for each day for 2 weeks
	  ○ Students reported improvements in optimism, gratitude, and life satisfaction
	• Froh et al,[45] 2009
	  ○ 3rd, 8th, and 12th graders wrote and delivered a gratitude letter to someone important to them
	  ○ Low-affect students reported increased gratitude after intervention

Interventions that focus on Serenity	• Broderick and Metz,[19] 2009
	  ○ Seniors at a Catholic high school took part in a 6-lesson mindfulness curriculum
	  ○ Students reported increased calmness, relaxation, and self-acceptance as well as decreased negative affect
	• Huppert and Johnson,[46] 2010
	  ○ 14- to 15-year-old boys took part in a 4-lesson, 4-wk mindfulness course
	  ○ No significant difference in well-being or resilience
	• Elder et al,[47] 2011
	  ○ Used transcendental meditation
	  ○ Middle school students engaged in a 12-min mindfulness session at the start and end of the school day for 3 mo
	  ○ Students were calmer, happier, less hyperactive, and had increased focus
	  ○ Students also had increased scores in math and English over 1 y

Interventions that focus on Resilience	• Seligman et al,[13] 2009
	  ○ Used Penn Resiliency Program (PRP)
	  ○ PRP teaches cognitive reframing, relaxation, coping skills, and creative brainstorming
	  ○ Reviewed 17 studies and 2000 students
	  ○ PRP reduced symptoms of depression and anxiety, with significant, long-lasting effects to well-being
	• Bernard and Walton,[48] 2011
	  ○ Used You Can Do It program
	  ○ Teaches resilience, confidence, persistence, and organization
	  ○ Compared fifth grade students in public schools
	  ○ Over 1 y, students had significant improvements in morale, connectedness, motivation, and behavior

(continued on next page)

Table 1 (continued)	
Intervention	**Applications and Program Descriptions**

Interventions that focus on Character Strengths	• Austin (2005)[49]
	  ○ Used Gallop Strengths Framework
	  ○ Completed Gallop Strengths Finder to highlight individual strengths, then shared these strengths with friends and family
	  ○ Students had significantly higher self-efficacy, expectations, extrinsic motivation, self-empowerment, and perceptions of ability
	• Seligman et al[13] (2009)
	  ○ Used Strath Haven Positive Psychology Program (SPPP)
	  ○ SPPP teaches skills for creating positive emotion
	  ○ Ninth grade students in language art class participated in positive psychology curriculum
	  ○ Students reported greater enjoyment and engagement
	• Madden et al,[50] 2011
	  ○ Used Values in Action-based coaching program
	  ○ VIA tests character strengths
	  ○ Fifth grade boys at private school wrote letters to their future selves highlighting character strengths and goals
	  ○ Students reported increased hope and engagement

Data from Waters L. A review of school-based positive psychology interventions. Australia Educ Dev Psychologist 2011;28(2):75–90.

limitations. Mindfulness, for example, is easy to teach at the basic level and can be learned and potentially applied by the student anywhere at any time. Although mindfulness' mental health benefits are increasingly appreciated,[15] especially for nonclinically referred student populations, CBT-based practices tend to provide the strongest reduction in actual symptoms, although requiring significant training to teach and practice effectively.

When it comes to outcomes, many interventions that are resilience based or focus on positive youth development (eg, the Developmental Assets Framework; www.search-institute.org/) have shown promise. Although effect sizes vary between studies, the interventions have been successful in reducing symptoms of specific mental health conditions like depression and anxiety,[16] as well as promoting overall improvements in morale, motivation, confidence, and connectedness.[17,18]

Broderick and Metz,[19] for example, tested a program called *Learn to Breathe*, which made use of 30- to 40-minute sessions 2 times a week, for 5 weeks. It resulted in both a significant decrease in negative affect and a significant increase in positive affect. Suldo and colleagues[20] implemented a 10-week *Well-Being Promotion Program*, a comprehensive, school-based PPI that showed steady improvements in sixth graders' life satisfaction over the course of the program. This program is based heavily on Seligman's[21] framework for improving happiness and well-being in adulthood and includes both core sessions' instructions and the specific worksheets a school practitioner could use when implementing this program. **Table 2** provides an overview of core sessions in the Well-Being Promotion Program for Groups of Adolescents.

Well-being curricula such as mindfulness programs require a significant amount of planning and organization before implementation. Gould and colleagues[22] propose 5 recommendations to facilitate the incorporation of school-based mindfulness programs. First, programs should define their core components and ideas for any given program. Second, ideas should be clearly articulated, especially to the students. Third, programs should also be able to report multiple dimensions of the fidelity of their intervention (FOI), like dosage, adherence, quality, and responsiveness. Fourth, they should develop accurate measures of their FOI to establish accuracy and precision. Finally, a common framework of FOIs should be established to facilitate communication between programs and schools. Such efforts to measure well-being educational programs can help improve the overall database needed to establish the effectiveness of these activities and the mechanisms that lie behind the positive changes that are observed.

As Suldo[1] points out, the focus of well-being research is moving from subjective well-being to the PERMA and modified PERMA models described in Seligman[23] and Kern and colleagues.[24] With the growing diversity of the youth that clinicians serve in school-based settings, cultural considerations in the assessment of well-being become even more important. For example, whereas achievement-oriented youth who are raised in white suburban cultures may embrace specific practices to develop "personal happiness," more relationally oriented youth may have values favoring development of happiness more focused on social connections.

EDUCATOR CONSIDERATIONS

Teachers play a crucial role in promoting the overall health and academic engagement of their students, in addition to their social and emotional learning and development. As McCullough and colleagues[25] have highlighted:

> Without a more direct focus on teacher well-being, the proposed strategies for promoting youth happiness may be futile, especially if the adults with whom they interact with most during the school day feel emotionally exhausted and overworked. Accordingly, Hills and Robinson emphasized that teachers need to be the first to put on their oxygen masks prior to supporting their students' social-emotional wellness.[26(pp.104)]

Other research has shown that a student's relationships with various parties (teachers, parents, and therapists) imply a set of secondary relationships among those parties.[27] These relationships are included under a *supporting alliance* that can help to buffer the everyday stressors that teachers may experience in the work with an educationally diverse group of learners. A strong supporting alliance can help teachers feel support and engender a sense that they work as part of a proverbial "village" that helps to educate students. This alliance can help prevent compassion fatigue, burnout, and attrition among teachers.

COLLEGE AND UNIVERSITY

Numerous courses have now been implemented in colleges and universities to promote happiness and well-being. At Yale, for example, "The Science of Well-Being" reviews what psychological research says about happiness and assigns students to put those strategies into practice. At Stanford, the "Psychology of Stoked" course is

Table 2
Overview of core sessions in the well-being promotion program for small groups of adolescents

Session	Target	Strategies	Comments
1	Positive introduction	You at your best	Students write about a time when they were at their best, then share and reflect on their personal strengths that were relevant
2	Gratitude (positive emotions about the past, I)	Gratitude journal	Used as a means of focusing on things, people, and events for which they are thankful
3	Gratitude (positive emotions about the past, II)	Gratitude journal reflection, and gratitude visit	Journal entrees are shared (matched to participants' comfort level); introduction of enacting gratitude through visits; connections made among thoughts, feelings, and actions
4	Kindness (positive emotions about the present)	Acts of kindness	Students introduced to kindness as a strength and asked to perform 5 acts of kindness during one designated day per week; specific acts of kindness are shared and suggested as examples
5	Character strengths I (positive emotions about the present)	Introduction to Strengths through VIA modeling	Students recount and share some of the kind acts they completed. Such retelling provides a method of active "savoring" of these experiences; students learn to define and recognize each of the 24 character strengths (VIA classification system); revisiting the "You at your best" activity to identify personal strengths displayed in their stories; based on their self-awareness and input by peers or others, they try and guess what their signature strengths may be

(continued on next page)

Table 2
(continued)

Session	Target	Strategies	Comments
6	Character strengths II (positive emotions about the present)	Survey assessment of signature character strengths	Students complete the online VIA youth survey before the session; in session, the practitioner helps each student (a) review the computer-generated report that lists and describes their character strengths, (b) identify their signature strengths, and (c) select one signature strength to use in a new way, each day, for 1 wk
7	Character strengths III (positive emotions about the present); savoring	Use of signature strengths in new ways; learn savoring methods	Introduces concept of using strengths across key domains of life; focus is on school, friendships, and family
8	Optimistic thinking (positive emotions about the future)	Optimistic explanatory style	Students are helped to consider ways they think about the various good and bad things in their lives, and why they may have happened; specific examples of optimistic explanatory styles (vs negative styles) are shared by the practitioner
9	Hope	Best-possible self in the future	Students visualize and write about their best possible future selves, including ways they will reach their specific goals
10	All	Transition/termination; review of strategies and plan for future uses	Begins with prior session, by reviewing homework with student accomplishments, and celebration of success of students' practice of positive psychology exercises

From Suldo SM, Savage JA, Mercer SH. Increasing middle school students' life satisfaction: efficacy of a positive psychology group intervention. J Happiness Stud 2014;15(1):28–30; with permission.

offered as an introductory seminar for freshmen and sophomores and reviews seminal work on the biological, psychological, cultural, and social aspects of well-being. The course teaches well-being theory from multiple points of view, including neuroscience, psychology, spirituality, and philosophy. Numerous in-class and out-of-class activities also challenge the learner to rethink assumptions on personal happiness.

At New York University and the University of Vermont, their "Science of Happiness" course examines the state of college student mental health and wellness on both a personal and a systems level. The instructors invite participants to reevaluate their beliefs, values, and assumptions about happiness and well-being and highlight key findings from positive psychology and the study of mental illness. At both of these universities, the class is part of a minor a student can take in Child and Adolescent Mental Health Studies (New York University) or Behavioral Change (University of Vermont).

MEDICAL SCHOOL

Medical schools are increasingly aware that educating students about well-being and health promotion benefits not only the future patients of these students but also the students themselves.[28] From research such as the landmark studies of adverse child experiences (ACEs) and the foundation of behavioral health for all health,[29] medical school curricula are allocating more time to educate students about the many ways that behavior and psychological health play crucial roles in the development and maintenance of disease morbidity and mortality.[30,31] In 2004, the Institute of Medicine published an authoritative report recommending improvements in the teaching of social and behavioral determinants of health.[32] Significant progress in this area has occurred, and although there remains continued room for improvement, research demonstrates that social and behavioral topics are discussed with patients on attending rounds during which medical students are often present.[33] More comprehensive teaching in areas such as nutrition, exercise, substance use, sleep, and other areas related to well-being is also taking place, not only in traditional lecture formats but also by using more interactive platforms, such as small-group discussions, case-based presentations, and patient simulations, that allow students to hone their skills in being able to apply this knowledge when talking to patients.[34,35]

Responding to data that continue to show high levels of stress, suicidality, and burnout among medical students,[36] many medical schools have also implemented well-being programs targeted for students themselves. These projects often involve combinations of changes to the medical school curriculum and procedures in ways that may alleviate stress (such as using pass/fail grading) and/or the introduction of specific wellness practices, such as mindfulness-based stress reduction. Many of these efforts have been successful in getting students to participate in these activities and in reducing levels of anxiety and depression.[37,38]

RESIDENCY AND FELLOWSHIP

In 2014, a committee sponsored by the Accreditation Council for Graduate Medical Education (ACGME) and the American Board of Psychiatry and Neurology published a standard set of educational objectives that would be required for all trainees across all accredited institutions in the United States. Before this time, requirements existed for residents and fellows to do certain rotations (eg, inpatient psychiatry), but the specific content related to what knowledge, skills, and attitudes trainees needed to have was not specified. All medical specialties were required to do this for their training programs, and these requirements are referred to as "milestones" to reflect various levels of competence on a particular area as one progresses through their training. In child psychiatry, there are 21 different milestones. One of those with regard to medical knowledge, MK3, specifies that child psychiatry trainees need to be proficient in their medical knowledge of both psychopathology and wellness. Although these milestones are often viewed as technicalities, the practical reality is that, since 2014, education not only about psychiatric illness but also about well-being is now a supported and required component of postgraduate training in child psychiatry.

These milestones, however, lack clarification about exactly *how* a training program best prepares the next generation of child psychiatrists to become proficient in well-being and its application to clinical care. At the child psychiatry training program at the University of Vermont, a didactic seminar was created called "Positive Child Psychiatry and Wellness" that covered the science and practical applications of many of the topics addressed in this issue.[39] Soon, other fellowship programs became interested in offering the seminar to their own fellows and contributed teaching resources that reflected their own areas of expertise. Beginning in 2017, the seminar started to be offered online though videoconferencing technology to the Georgetown and New York University child fellowship programs as well, cotaught in real time by faculty at all 3 institutions and McLean Hospital in Boston, Massachusetts. A pretest and posttest that included clinical vignettes were also done, with preliminary results showing gains in knowledge for wellness topics but not significant changes in clinical approach among child psychiatry fellows.[40]

Such a result was not unexpected and underscores the need to advance beyond lectures to produce measurable changes in a young psychiatrist's clinical behavior. Successful training of psychiatry residents and child psychiatrists in the science of well-being and the application of that science to practice appears to require simultaneous efforts in 3 main areas, as follows:

1. Didactic instruction
2. Supervision with attention to well-being practices integrated into evaluations and treatment plans
3. Clinic infrastructure and culture.

Each of these pillars is discussed in turn and is also summarized in **Table 3**.

The didactic component was previously mentioned in the example of specific seminars that cover many aspects of well-being. These seminars are important to provide, because it is not sufficient to suggest that the simple absence of negative developmental factors is enough for optimal brain development. For example, the negative effects of ACEs are now well established, but knowledge about ACEs is incomplete without also understanding how the *presence* of positive factors, such as parental warmth, can enhance development and protect against psychopathology.[41] These didactic components are also valuable in helping trainees understand the evidence base behind many of the activities and techniques that are encouraged.

Much of this information learned in these sessions can also serve a dual role with regards to the Common Program Requirements from the ACGME that now mandate programmatic attention to the mental health and well-being of the trainees themselves. For those unfamiliar with this new set of training requirements, these refer to efforts that the program must now do to help mitigate against the increasingly recognized problem of physician burnout and to promote levels of professional engagement, resilience, and enthusiasm.[42] Specific attention to how trainees can apply these principles individually can be useful in helping trainees not only to engage their patients about these topics but also to help them "walk the walk" in their own lives.

The supervision component in training is also critical, especially in helping trainees incorporate what they have learned about wellness and health promotion to their routine interactions with patients and families. Consider, for example, a child psychiatrist supervisor as a fellow presents a case about a patient being evaluated for attention-deficit/hyperactivity disorder. If the supervisor focuses primarily on *Diagnostic and Statistical Manual of Mental Disorders, Fifth Edition* criteria and medication

| Table 3 |
| Comprehensive teaching of well-being to psychiatric trainees |

Elements of Well-Being Education in Psychiatry Residency and Fellowships	
Didactics	Specific seminars directed at topics, such as happiness, well-being, wellness activities, and positive parenting, that reflect the current state of knowledge and practical techniques that help trainees incorporate this knowledge into practice
Supervision	Requiring trainees during supervision to assess and focus on well-being in their assessment and treatments providing guidance on how to make these elements part of routine care
Infrastructure	Providing trainees the time and the tools, such as rating scales or other assessment instruments, that allow for the efficient gathering of information about family-based wellness and health promotion and their emphasis in follow-up appointments

history, it is likely that important history regarding physical activity, screen time, bedtime routines, and nutrition will not be obtained, thereby closing off important potential avenues for intervention relevant for children with attention problems and hyperactivity. On the other hand, supervision that conveys the expectation that trainees need to be knowledgeable about these areas of family functioning in order to use them in their treatment plans will enhance these elements becoming a routine part of a trainee's approach to patient care.

The likelihood of being able to gather and use information about well-being is also greatly enhanced if the culture of the clinic values it and reflects that valuation in its infrastructure. One specific example of this culture would be in having intake forms and rating scales that include questions about well-being and health behaviors. It also includes building a clinic that allows the clinicians the time and space to address these issues with families. If a fellow, for example, is expected to perform a well-being informed follow-up appointment within the confines of a 15-minute "medication management" visit (a term that should be considered for retirement), it will be very difficult for that fellow to make even thoughtful pharmacologic decisions, let alone recommendations about well-being and health promotion. In the many instances when the treatment of a child and family members is split between multiple different clinicians, the clinic environment also needs to support and encourage communication between them to maximize the level of coordination.

When these pillars of didactic training, supervision, and infrastructure all include attention to patient and family well-being, trainees have the highest potential to view wellness and health promotion as simply what psychiatrists do. As these trainees graduate and enter the workforce, this perspective will help propel the entire field to broaden the expertise to where it belongs, namely, the entire continuum of mental health.

SUMMARY

Although more explicit teaching on well-being and the techniques to promote it remain underutilized at all levels of learning, there has been an increase of late in wellness-oriented education that shows promise in helping individuals improve their levels of emotional-behavioral health. At the elementary, middle, and high school levels, many programs and curricula now exist that have demonstrated efficacy in promoting positive traits and coping strategies. In colleges across the country and beyond, courses about wellness and happiness are becoming increasingly popular not only because of their intellectual content but also due to their many practical benefits that students can incorporate into their own lives. When it comes to medical training, institutions are recognizing the importance for both well-being of the students themselves and those students' future benefits of content that reflects how foundational emotional-behavioral well-being is to overall health. Psychiatric residencies and child psychiatry fellowships are also attempting to augment their rigorous training of psychopathology with additional education on well-being and the factors that actively promote positive brain development. These efforts show promise in equipping the next generation of psychiatrists to be true mental health professionals with knowledge and expertise that can help their patients not only to relieve symptoms but also to realize their full human potential.

REFERENCES

1. Suldo SM. Promoting student happiness: positive psychology interventions in schools. New York: Guilford Press; 2016.
2. O'Grady P. Positive psychology in the elementary school classroom. New York: W.W. Norton & Company; 2013.
3. Joshi SV, Lenoir L, Ojakian M, et al. K12 mental health promotion and suicide prevention toolkit. 2017. Available at http://www.heardalliance.org/toolkit-promotion-sel/. Accessed October 7, 2018.
4. Merikangas KR, He JP, Burstein M, et al. Lifetime prevalence of mental disorders in U.S. adolescents: results from the National Comorbidity survey Replication–Adolescent Supplement (NCS-A). J Am Acad Child Adolesc Psychiatry 2010; 49:980–9.
5. CDC. Youth online: high school YRBA - United States Results 2017. Available at: https://nccd.cdc.gov/YouthOnline/App/Results.aspx?LID=XX. Accessed August 20, 2018.
6. Furlong MJ, You S, Renshaw TL, et al. Preliminary development and validation of the social and emotional health survey for secondary school students. Soc Indic Res 2014;117:1011–32.
7. Furlong MJ, You S, Renshaw TL, et al. Preliminary development of the positive experiences at school scale for elementary school children. Child Indic Res 2013;6: 753–75.
8. Furlong MJ, Dowdy E, Carnazzo K, et al. Covitality: fostering the building blocks of complete mental health. NASP Communiqué 2014;42(8):27–8.
9. Suldo SM, Huebner ES. Does life satisfaction moderate the effects of stressful life events on psychopathological behavior during adolescence? Sch Psychol Q 2004;19:93–105.
10. Suldo SM, Shaffer EJ. Looking beyond psychopathology: the dual factor model of mental health in youth. Sch Psychol Rev 2008;37:52–68.
11. Stiglbauer B, Gnambs T, Gamsjager M, et al. The upward spiral of adolescents' positive school experiences and happiness: investigating reciprocal effects over time. J Sch Psychol 2013;51:231–42.
12. Waters L. A review of school-based positive psychology interventions. Aust Educ Dev Psychol 2011;28:75–90.
13. Seligman MEP, Ernst RM, Gillham J, et al. Positive education: positive psychology and classroom interventions. Oxford Rev Education 2009;35:293–311.
14. Durlak JA, Weissberg RP, Dymnicki AB, et al. The impact of enhancing students' social and emotional learning: a meta-analysis of school-based universal interventions. Child Dev 2011;82:405–32.

15. Keng SL, Smoski MJ, Robins CJ. Effects of mindfulness on psychological health: a review of empirical studies. Clin Psychol Rev 2011;31:1041–56.
16. Dray J, Bowman J, Wolfenden L, et al. Systematic review of universal resilience interventions targeting child and adolescent mental health in the school setting: review protocol. Syst Rev 2015;4:186.
17. Zoogman S, Goldberg SB, Hoyt WT, et al. Mindfulness interventions with youth: a meta-analysis. Mindfulness (N Y) 2015;6:290–302.
18. Dunning DL, Griffiths K, Kuyken W, et al. The effects of mindfulness-based interventions on cognition and mental health in children and adolescents: a meta-analysis of randomised controlled trials. 2018. Available at: https://doi.org/10.31234/osf.io/rj5mk. Accessed October 5, 2018.
19. Broderick PC, Metz S. Learning to breathe: a pilot trial of a mindfulness curriculum for adolescents. Adv Sch Ment Health Promot 2009;2:35–46.
20. Suldo SM, Savage JA, Mercer S. Increasing middle-school students' life satisfaction: efficacy of a positive psychology group intervention. J Happiness Stud 2014;15:19–42.
21. Seligman MEP. Authentic happiness: using the new positive psychology to realize your potential for lasting fulfillment. New York: Free Press; 2002.
22. Gould LF, Dariotis JK, Greenberg MT, et al. Assessing fidelity of implementation (FOI) for school-based mindfulness and yoga Interventions: a systematic review. Mindfulness (N Y) 2016;7:5–33.
23. Seligman MEP. Flourish: a visionary new understanding of happiness and well-being. New York: Free Press; 2011.
24. Kern ML, Waters LE, Adler A, et al. A multidimensional approach to measuring well-being in students: application of the PERMA framework. J Posit Psychol 2015;10:262–71.
25. McCullough M, Quinlan D. Universal Strategies for Promoting Student Happiness. In: Suldo SM, editor. Promoting Student Happiness: Positive Psychology Interventions in Schools. New York, NY: Guilford Press; 2016. p. 103–21.
26. Hills KJ, Robinson A. Enhancing teacher well-being: put on your oxygen masks! Communique 2010;39:1–17.
27. Feinstein NF, Fielding K, Udvari-Solner A, et al. The supporting alliance in child and adolescent treatment: enhancing collaboration between therapists, parents and teachers. Am J Psychother 2009;63:319–44.
28. Association of American Medical Colleges. Behavioral and social science foundations for future physicians: report of the behavioral and social science expert panel. 2011. Available at: https://www.aamc.org/download/271020/data/behavioralandsocialsciencefoundationsforfuturephysicians.pdf. Accessed October 1, 2018.
29. Felitti VJ, Anda RF, Nordenberg D, et al. Relationship of childhood abuse and household dysfunction to many of the leading causes of death in adults. The Adverse Childhood Experiences (ACE) Study. Am J Prev Med 1998;14:245–58.
30. Farouk A. Rethinking how physicians learn to prevent, manage chronic disease. Chicago, IL: AMA Wire; 2016.
31. Mokdad AH, Marks JS, Stroup DF, et al. Actual causes of death in the United States, 2000. JAMA 2004;291:1238–45.
32. Institute of Medicine. Improving medical education: enhancing the social and behavioral science content of medical school curricula. Washington, DC: National Academy Press; 2004.
33. Satterfield JM, Bereknyei S, Hilton JF, et al. The prevalence of social and behavioral topics and related educational opportunities during attending rounds. Acad Med 2014;89:1548–57.

34. Satterfield JM, Mitteness LS, Tervalon M, et al. Integrating the social and behavioral sciences in an undergraduate medical curriculum: the UCSF essential core. Acad Med 2004;79(1):6–15.
35. Post DM, Stone LC, Knutson DJ, et al. Enhancing behavioral science education at the Ohio State University College of Medicine. Acad Med 2008;83:28–36.
36. Dyrbye LN, Thomas MR, Shanafelt TD. Systematic review of depression, anxiety, and other indicators of psychological distress among U.S. and Canadian medical students. Acad Med 2006;81:354–73.
37. Slavin SJ, Schindler DL, Chibnall JT. Medical student mental health 3.0: improving student wellness through curricular changes. Acad Med 2014;89: 573–7.
38. Drolet BC, Rodgers S. A comprehensive medical student wellness program–design and implementation at Vanderbilt School of Medicine. Acad Med 2010; 85:103–10.
39. Rettew DC, Althoff RR, Hudziak JJ. Happy kids: teaching trainees about emotional-behavioral wellness, not just illness. Poster presented a the 43rd Annual Conference of the American Association of Directors in Psychiatric Residency Training in Tucson, AZ, March 13-15, 2014.
40. Rettew DC, Schlechter A, Bostic J, et al. A shared videoconferenced didactic seminar in positive child psychiatry across unaffiliated fellowship programs. Poster presented at the 47th annual meeting of the American Association of Directors in Psychiatry Residency Training in New Orleans, LA, March 1-3, 2018.
41. Carroll JE, Gruenewald TL, Taylor SE, et al. Childhood abuse, parental warmth, and adult multisystem biological risk in the coronary artery risk development in Young Adults Study. Proc Natl Acad Sci U S A 2013;110:17149–53.
42. Gengoux GW, Roberts LW. Enhancing wellness and engagement among healthcare professionals. Acad Psychiatry 2018;42:1–4.
43. Marques SC, Pais-Ribeiro JL, Lopez SJ. The role of positive psychology constructs in predicting mental health and academic achievement in children and adolescents: a two-year longitudinal study. J Happiness Stud 2011;12:1049–62.
44. Froh JJ, Sefick WJ, Emmons RA. Counting blessings in early adolescents: An experimental study of gratitude and subjective well-being. Journal of School Psychology 2008;46:213–33.
45. Froh JJ, Kashdan TB, Ozimkowski KM, et al. Who benefits the most from a gratitude intervention in children and adolescents? examining positive affect as a moderator. J Pos Psychology 2009;4:408–22.
46. Huppert FA, Johnson DM. A controlled trial of mindfulness training in schools: the importance of practice for an impact on well-being. J Pos Psychology 2010;5: 264–74.
47. Elder C, Nidich S, Colbert R, et al. Reduced psychological distress in racial and ethnic minority students practicing the transcendental meditation program. J Instruct Psychology 2011;38:109–16.
48. Bernard PME, Walton K. The effect of you can do it! education in six schools on student perceptions of well-being, teaching-learning and relationships. J Student Wellbeing 2011;5:22–37.
49. Austin D. The effects of a strengths development intervention program upon the self-perception of students' academic abilities. Dissertation Abstracts International 2005;66:1631A.
50. Madden W, Green S, Grant AM. A pilot study evaluating strengths-based coaching for primary school students: enhancing engagement and hope. International Coaching Psychology Review 2011;6:71–83.

Where Do We Go from Here? Additional Opportunities to Address Well-Being in Child Psychiatry Clinical Practice and Advocacy for Children and Families

Emily Aron, MD[a],*, Matthew G. Biel, MD, MSc[a,b]

KEYWORDS

- Well-being • Technology • Resilience • Consultation • Family • Telepsychiatry

KEY POINTS

- Child psychiatrists should play an active role in helping parents and children to develop healthy media use habits.
- Child psychiatrists can use technology including mobile applications and telepsychiatry to enhance clinical care.
- Strength-based approaches build patient engagement and enhance outcomes in assessment and treatment in child psychiatry.
- Strength-based approaches and interventions that target well-being can enhance child psychiatrists work with parents as well in consultation with schools and other community settings.

INTRODUCTION

The preceding articles of this issue have outlined emergent research findings, promising clinical strategies, and novel programming efforts that incorporate the science of well-being into child and adolescent psychiatry. This concluding article formulates a response to the following questions: "Where do we go from here? What are additional considerations that can be included in clinical practice now and in the near

Disclosure Statement: None.
[a] Department of Psychiatry, Medstar Georgetown University Hospital, Georgetown University Medical Center, 2115 Wisconsin Avenue Northwest, Washington, DC 20007, USA; [b] Department of Pediatrics, Medstar Georgetown University Hospital, Georgetown University Medical Center, 3800 Reservoir Rd NW, Washington, DC 20007, USA
* Corresponding author.
E-mail address: emilyaron@gmail.com

Child Adolesc Psychiatric Clin N Am 28 (2019) 281–288
https://doi.org/10.1016/j.chc.2018.11.012
1056-4993/19/© 2018 Elsevier Inc. All rights reserved.

childpsych.theclinics.com

future that might build upon this emerging evidence and clinical wisdom? How can child and adolescent psychiatrists and other mental health professionals best advocate for this new science of well-being to support children and families?" Preceding articles have illuminated relevant information and strategies to incorporate research findings related to nutrition, exercise, mindfulness, and a well-being–focused approach to the clinical practice of child psychiatry. Additional considerations that are gaining traction and importance in clinical care follow here.

PROMOTING HEALTHY USE OF MEDIA AND TECHNOLOGY

Technology has dramatically changed the way that children and families communicate, recreate, and learn over the first 2 decades of the twenty-first century. The ubiquity of Internet access through mobile devices has been particularly powerful in its impact on children and parents, and the potential for overuse of digital media has generated appropriate concern.[1] Social media in particular is drawing enormous attention for potential negative impact on adolescents. However, these tools also present opportunities to deliver positive messaging and to promote well-being. Youth access the Internet and social media as a way to both seek help and communicate their suffering.[1–3] Clinicians benefit from a curious and engaged stance toward technology in their work with children and families. This stance promotes considering strategies to mitigate negative impact of excessive media exposure, while at the same time promoting select use of technology-based tools that promote well-being and enhance social support.

Although excessive use of the Internet and digital media is associated with negative physical and mental health outcomes for children and adolescents, there is a plethora of content available to help engage this age group with well-being. For example, numerous smartphone applications have emerged that allow individuals to participate in mindfulness exercises (commonly used examples that have free versions include *Stop, Breathe and Think*; *Calm;* and *Headspace*). Physical exercise trackers are increasingly popular and encourage youth to exercise and stay physically active (eg, Fitbit and the Apple iPhone and iWatch). Biofeedback apps allow individuals to track their physiology such as heart rate and implement cognitive and behavioral exercises to help reach a state of calm or relaxation (eg, HeartMath and Spire). Emerging research is measuring the impact of these technologies as a part of clinical practice, and clinicians can take advantage of these resources, both for themselves and for their patients, in promoting well-being practices.

In clinical practice, incorporating therapeutic uses of technology creates an opportunity to discuss health media practices within a family. In response to an increase in concern regarding digital media consumption and lack of guidelines, the American Academy of Pediatrics developed the Family Media Use Plan (www.healthychildren.org/MediaUsePlan), an interactive checklist based on the developmental age of a child. It encourages the family to discuss media use together and also highlights the need for parents to role model healthy media use and etiquette. As more children and adolescents become fluent with technology and use it for their own purposes, so too do their parents. There is a growing need to monitor how technology is shaping the mental health of youth and their families in a broader ecological context. As a start, child psychiatrists can assess media use during initial assessments through the use of a general questionnaire or as a point of general interest and concern. Following the evaluation, clinicians can provide tools such as the Family Media Use Plan to set parameters in collaboration with the child and family.

One specific strategy that uses technological advances to address mental health concerns in children and families is the practice of telepsychiatry.[4] The scarcity and skewed distribution of child and adolescent psychiatrists across the United States directly affects the well-being of youth with psychopathology, particularly those who have additional psychosocial risk factors including poverty and reduced access to health care. Adopting telepsychiatry practices within child psychiatry can positively affect the well-being of children with less access to care. Benefits of a clinical care delivery model that incorporates telepsychiatry include the following:

1. Meeting families and children "where they are."
2. Reducing the demands placed on families, such as travel expenses and time traveling to a clinic.
3. Providing more flexibility for clinicians as to when and where they provide care.
4. Decreasing time away from school, home, and/or work for children and families.
5. Engaging youth through the use of technology in a comfortable and familiar setting.

PROMOTING STRENGTHS IN CLINICAL ASSESSMENT AND TREATMENT

Psychiatry, as a medical discipline, approaches clinical diagnosis of mental illness and treatment of related symptoms through a disease-based or deficit lens. Adopting a strength-based focus in the clinical setting is an alternative to traditional psychiatry practice. A strength-based approach balances inquiry into negative attributes and symptoms of a disorder with an effort to highlight strengths and assets that can promote growth in the context of adversity. This alternative paradigm shifts the clinical focus from sole focus on diagnosing and treating mental illness to recognizing strengths and aiming for mental health recovery. Within this approach, mental health issues are destigmatized and seen as a common aspect of everyday life. An individual's unique set of abilities is then identified as the key to improving functioning and having a life that is fulfilling.

The article on "The Positive Assessment: A Model for Integrating Well-Being and Strengths-Based Approaches into the Child and Adolescent Psychiatry Clinical Evaluation" by Schlechter and colleagues in this issue details the rationale and strategies for prioritizing positive emotions and positive attributes within clinical interviews and treatment in child psychiatry. These approaches have promising supporting evidence, among general populations of youth as well as among youth with significantly impairing psychiatric illness, suggesting that these strategies are relevant for mental health promotion and prevention as well as for recovery from mental illness, and should not be limited to work with high-functioning or "worried well" children. Looking at a large epidemiologic sample of children and adolescents in the general population in England, Vidal-Ribas and colleagues[5] demonstrated via a path analytical model that positive attributes of children as reported by parents predicted less psychiatric disturbance at baseline and at 3-year follow-up. In the absence of mental illness, this study suggests that positive attributes are protective in preventing clinically significant psychiatric problems. Among a clinical population, Lyons and colleagues[6] demonstrated that children living in a residential treatment center who have higher level of strengths are more likely to have a positive disposition outcome (ie, return home) and those with fewer strengths were more likely to have a negative disposition outcome (ie, detention, hospital). The investigators also demonstrated that individual strengths were inversely correlated with functional impairment, independent of symptom severity. The study highlights that youth with significant mental illness may also possess significant strengths that can alter their life trajectories. In a related study with severely psychiatrically ill youth, patients who identified strengths and then developed coping skills based on these strengths and practiced them over the period of an inpatient hospitalization were found to have higher scores on self-efficacy and self-esteem.[7] Given the chronic nature of mental illness, the improvement of overall functioning by focusing on improving a person's resources, assets, and skills is vital in the field of child psychiatry.

These findings suggest that a strength-based approach may have a key role in child and adolescent psychiatric practice. Training programs can integrate the focus on assets and positive attributes in concert with traditional didactics focusing on symptoms and psychopathology. Focusing on strengths in the clinical encounter provides an opportunity for clinicians to form therapeutic alliances with patients who are less motivated and less engaged in treatment. This dynamic may be of particular relevance in treating children and families from underserved groups such as racial, ethnic, and sexual minorities, who are less likely to access effective mental health care as a result of complex factors including stigma, inequitable allocation of clinical resources, and previous negative experiences with mental health providers. By shifting the focus from what is wrong with an individual to what is going well, child psychiatrists can contribute to the recovery process from a standpoint of humility, curiosity, and optimism.

PROMOTING HEALTHY FAMILIES

The apple may or may not fall far from a tree; however, it is undeniable that the tree is essential in shaping the apple wherever it may land. Children are inextricably linked to their family environs and, as clinicians, nurturing that fertile ground is an important task. Links between parent psychopathology and child psychopathology are complex, bidirectional, and critically important in clinical outcomes for both generations.[8,9] Family support and relationships are critical factors in understanding risk and resilience in the setting of childhood adversity and trauma.[10] Supporting children's positive attributes from a strength- and resilience-based approach will yield better results when parents are also capable of being present and supportive of their children. Addressing the mental health of families and enhancing their wellness can further serve as a way to connect with families in the office and engage them in treatment. Offering support to parents and providing alternatives to current parenting practices, rather than admonishing them for parenting failures or leaving them out of treatment altogether, models how they can similarly support their struggling offspring in addition to promoting their own sense of self-efficacy and well-being.

There is an urgent need for clinical strategies that more actively address family strengths and vulnerabilities as a core component of child and adolescent psychiatric care. One example of such an approach is the Vermont Family-Based Approach (VFBA), which dedicates resources toward both the well-being of children and their caregivers. The article on "Health Promotion in Primary Care Pediatrics: Initial Results of the Randomized Controlled Trial of the Vermont Family Based Approach" by Ivanova and colleagues in this issue describes the results of applying this approach in a pediatric primary care setting, highlighting a promising direction for the role that child psychiatry can play in integrated care strategies that are family focused. In a recent issue of this series, the same investigators describe the VFBA in an outpatient child psychiatry setting.[11] The clinic conducts a rigorous assessment of the family using rating scales completed by the child (about themselves and parents) and parents (about themselves and the child). Families where parents have clinically significant symptoms are placed in an "at-risk" group, meaning the child is at risk for psychopathology, given the family environment and parent functioning. This group receives support from a "coach" to address the emotional and behavioral health of the parents. When children are found to suffer from emotional or behavioral problems, they are categorized as "affected" and also receive a coach and work with a psychiatrist. The psychiatrist's role is also extended beyond providing medications and diagnoses. The psychiatrist helps to interpret the results of the family-based assessment, design and implement the family's program of health and wellness, and use preventive practices. Individual components of the program are supported by emerging research.[11]

Using the VFBA as a model, psychiatrists can incorporate tenets of well-being in their encounters with caregivers. The elements and research on well-being have been discussed in previous articles in this issue. This approach can be particularly helpful in building a constructive therapeutic relationship with parents. Focusing on elements of well-being (positive emotions, engagement, positive relationships, meaning, and accomplishment) as applied to parenting is helpful in reframing a potentially conflicted relationship between caregiver and child. The following are a few examples of questions that a clinician can ask parents:

1. Tell me about your proudest moment as a parent.
2. Has parenting affected your relationships? How?
3. Are there times when you feel time go by without noticing? Does that ever happen when you are with your child?
4. What do you and your child enjoy doing together?
5. What is most important to you right now? What do you prioritize?

These types of questions can shift the conversation with caregivers from one that is focused on what is going wrong with the child to exploring things that are going well. They can also bring the parent into the clinical picture without introducing blame, prescribing what the parent should be doing, or highlighting what the parent is doing incorrectly.

PROMOTING HEALTHY COMMUNITIES

Understanding the home and community within which a child grows and thrives as well as ways in which the environment impedes healthy development is a crucial data point for clinicians, and it highlights opportunities for child psychiatrists to be advocates for child and family well-being. Child psychiatrists can be essential allies for supporting strategies to build healthy communities. Schools, child welfare agencies, and juvenile justice and other facilities within the legal system are natural partners in promoting well-being for children in the environments where they live, learn, and work to recover from adverse experiences. Psychiatrists may interact with these entities through clinical consultation, ongoing clinical care, or organizational consultation. In each of these roles, psychiatrists can emphasize well-being strategies and strengths-based approaches to working with and understanding children and families. During clinical discussions, including strength-based recommendations can shape the way a school or residential program approaches a student's behavior and academic challenges. By highlighting positive emotions, impactful relationships, and opportunities for meaning-making and purpose, these recommendations can orient educators and school staff toward the power of well-being to shape outcomes for young people. Some basic principles of well-being that can be incorporated into child psychiatry consultation in a range of community settings are included in **Box 1**, and these should be communicated clearly to partners and collaborators in these settings.

School-based mental health services are growing in many parts of North America and represent an outstanding opportunity to reduce barriers to access to pediatric mental health care. These services often include clinical consultation or direct treatment services from child psychiatrists. Participation in clinical care in schools offers

---

Box 1
Key principles of well-being in child psychiatry consultation

- Focusing on youths' strengths and attributes is effective
  - Improves treatment engagement
  - Improves treatment outcomes
- Epigenetics research teaches us that our experiences shape our brains
  - Positive relationships, activities, and emotions build our brains
  - Adversity and sustained stress harm our brains
- Mental health symptoms are common
  - Most people have symptoms at some time in their lives
  - When symptoms are impairing, this often reflects environmental factors
- Psychiatric diagnoses in children occur along a spectrum from mild to severe
  - Good treatment reduces severity of symptoms
  - Positive relationships, activities, and emotions reduce severity as well
- Well-being approaches such as exercise, nutrition, and mindfulness work
  - Can be as effective as more "clinical" interventions
  - No side effects and highly acceptable to children and families
- Every treatment plans needs to include the following:
  - Strategies to build positive relationships, activities, and emotions
  - Well-being activities to supplement other clinical care

---

to child psychiatrists an outstanding opportunity to support and influence the full spectrum of mental health supports that many schools now provide. These supports involve a range of strategies, including universal instruction in social-emotional learning, typically drawing on well-established evidence-based curricula (excellent reviews of a range of these curricula are available at www.casel.org/); more targeted interventions for students considered to be at higher risk for emotional and behavioral health strategies[12]; and direct clinical services for children determined to require treatment. This tiered model of mental health promotion, prevention, and treatment represents an excellent example of a population-level strategy that emphasizes a resilience-building, strengths-based approach to addressing the emotional and behavioral well-being of all children. Child psychiatrists should familiarize themselves with local versions of these approaches being applied in schools and their communities, so as to support robust implementation, help in identifying gaps in promotion/prevention/treatment services, and contribute the unique expertise and perspective on childhood development and well-being. In addition, child psychiatrists can build relationships with mentoring programs, after-school activities and clubs, and youth athletic organizations. Forming relationships with these programs can facilitate meaningful connections between patients, families, and resources in their community that build well-being.

Because the problems that many children face are not "cured" by individual therapy and medication alone, child psychiatrists must reckon with environmental factors in children's lives that are often critical in determining prognosis. Having a presence and voice in communities through speaking engagements, publishing in local papers, participating in health clinics and/or fairs, visiting schools, and joining in after-school activities can help strengthen child psychiatrists' voices in shaping ecological forces that let children thrive. Child psychiatrists can develop assertive voices in encouraging community-wide initiatives to address common risk factors affecting children, including bullying, suicide, and the negative impacts of excessive social media use on youth. Evidence for the health impacts of so-called social determinants of health such as poverty, housing instability, food insecurity, and discrimination and racism continue to grow, and the impact of these determinants on mental health and well-being may be particularly pernicious. Child psychiatrists can join growing advocacy efforts to support social policies that buffer the impact of these health factors; advocacy opportunities exist at local, state, and national levels to support policy changes that show particular promise, such as improved access to high-quality early childcare and education and paid family leave laws.

This issue focuses on the promise of clinical strategies in child and adolescent psychiatry that build on growing interest in the science of well-being. This interest is supported by emerging evidence from a range of research approaches, including neuroimaging, genetics, developmental psychology, and clinical psychology and psychiatry. As clinicians explore the role for these health promotion, prevention, and intervention strategies in their practices, there is a clear need for robust clinical research efforts to answer key questions about the effectiveness of these approaches for clinical populations with a range of emotional and behavioral health concerns. These efforts will build the capacity of our field to prioritize holistic approaches to clinical care and to expand our "toolbox" beyond limited therapies to include integrated strategies that will enhance the well-being of all children.

REFERENCES

1. Hoge E, Bickham D, Cantor J. Digital media, anxiety, and depression in children. Pediatrics 2017;140(Suppl 2):S76–80.

2. Gould MS, Munfakh JL, Lubell K, et al. Seeking help from the internet during adolescence. J Am Acad Child Adolesc Psychiatry 2002;41(10):1182–9.

3. Trefflich F, Kalckreuth S, Mergl R, et al. Psychiatric patients' internet use corresponds to the internet use of the general public. Psychiatry Res 2015;226(1): 136–41.

4. American Academy of Child and Adolescent Psychiatry Clinical Update. Telepsychiatry with children and adolescents. J Am Acad Child Adolesc Psychiatry 2017; 56(10):875–93.

5. Vidal-Ribas P, Goodman R, Stringaris A. Positive attributes in children and reduced risk of future psychopathology. Br J Psychiatry 2015;206(1):17–25.

6. Lyons JS, Uziel-Miller ND, Reyes F, et al. Strengths of children and adolescents in residential settings: prevalence and associations with psychopathology and discharge placement. J Am Acad Child Adolesc Psychiatry 2000;39(2):176–81.

7. Toback RL, Graham-Bermann SA, Patel PD. Outcomes of a character strengths-based intervention on self-esteem and self-efficacy of psychiatrically hospitalized youths. Psychiatr Serv 2016;67(5):574–7.

8. Ungar M. Practitioner review: diagnosing childhood resilience–a systemic approach to the diagnosis of adaptation in adverse social and physical ecologies. J Child Psychol Psychiatry 2015;56(1):4–17.

9. Bayer JK, Morgan A, Prendergast LA, et al. Predicting temperamentally inhibited young children's clinical-level anxiety and internalizing problems from parenting and parent wellbeing: a population study. J Abnorm Child Psychol 2018;1–17.

10. Beardslee WR, Gladstone TR, Wright EJ, et al. A family-based approach to the prevention of depressive symptoms in children at risk: evidence of parental and child change. Pediatrics 2003;112(2):e119–31.

11. Hudziak J, Ivanova MY. The Vermont Family Based Approach: family based health promotion, illness prevention, and intervention. Child Adolesc Psychiatr Clin N Am 2016;25(2):167–78.

12. Jaycox LH, Langley A, Dean KL, et al. Making it easier for school staff to help traumatized students. Santa Monica (CA): RAND Corporation; 2009. Available at: https://www.rand.org/pubs/research_briefs/RB9443-1.html.